P9-CCR-349

VACCINES:

ARE THEY *REALLY* SAFE AND EFFECTIVE?

By Neil Z. Miller

New Atlantean Press
Santa Fe, New Mexico

VACCINES:
ARE THEY *REALLY* SAFE AND EFFECTIVE?

By Neil Z. Miller

All rights reserved. No part of this book may be reproduced, transmitted, or utilized in any form or by any means, electronic, photographic or mechanical, including photocopying, recording, or by any information storage and retrieval system, without written permission from the author, except for brief quotations in literary articles and reviews.

International Standard Book Number:
1-881217-30-2
Library of Congress Control Number:
2002103701

Copyright © 2002, 2004 by Neil Z. Miller

Cataloging-in-Publication Data
Miller, Neil Z.
   Vaccines : are they *really* safe and effective? /
by Neil Z. Miller
      p. cm.
   Includes bibliographical references and index.
   ISBN 1-881217-30-2
   1. Vaccination of children. 2. Immunization of children—
Complications—Risk factors and sequelae. 3. Communicable
diseases in children. 4. Vaccines—Health aspects. I. Title
614.47'083—dc21
                                                    2002103701

Cover photo: ImageState
Cover layout: Bill Pfau

Printed in the United States of America

Published by:
New Atlantean Press
PO Box 9638
Santa Fe, NM 87504

www.thinktwice.com

TABLE OF CONTENTS

Note: For information about the MMR vaccine, see the individual chapters on measles, mumps, and rubella. For DPT and DTaP, see the individual chapters on diphtheria, tetanus, pertussis, and acellular pertussis.

ACKNOWLEDGMENTS

I wish to acknowledge the following authors for their brave and pioneering accomplishments regarding vaccines: Hannah Allen, Harold Buttram, Harris Coulter, Barbara Loe Fisher, Walene James, Eleanor McBean, Robert S. Mendelsohn, and Richard Moskowitz. I also wish to express my appreciation to the many other unbiased vaccine researchers not mentioned here. For all of our children, thank you.

DISCLAIMER

The decision regarding whether or not to vaccinate is a personal one. The author is not a health practitioner nor legal advisor, and makes no claims in this regard. Nor does the author recommend for or against vaccines. All of the information in this book is taken from other sources and documented in the Notes. If you have questions, doubts, or concerns regarding any of the information in this book, go to the original source. Then research this topic even further so that you may make a wise and informed choice.

Foreword

George R. Schwartz, MD

I approached Neil Miller's book, *Vaccines: Are They Really Safe and Effective?*, with some trepidation, fearing a reckless diatribe against vaccination. My basic roots are in the traditional medical system, and I have advocated immunizations along the guidelines of the Centers for Disease Control (CDC). In fact, all of my children have received preventive immunizations. Yet, I have been aware of a growing movement within this country and other parts of the world toward questioning "routine" immunizations. By "routine" I mean the usual "baby shots," and not vaccines for particular high risk groups or for special occupations or travel. Certainly the smallpox vaccine is an example of one routine shot which was eventually discontinued when the morbidity (occurrence of the illness) from the immunization exceeded the benefits.

Into this controversy and fray, Mr. Miller has elected to enter. His is a passionate and articulate voice—one which cannot be dismissed easily. He has researched the subject extensively, and while I do not agree with some of his conclusions, I recognize that a new and intelligent voice has entered the arena.

Mr. Miller has used hundreds of references and he provides his sources. Although the tone of the book is occasionally extreme, it is clear when looking at the broader picture that Mr. Miller simply wants the best for his children and for other children as well. In his book, Mr. Miller questions routine immunizations. Therefore, his references tend toward the iconoclastic rather than the supportive variety in the medical literature. But his book is not an attempt at justifying existing practices, as by design it takes a strong stance in the anti-vaccination camp.

Why then should I—a physician who basically advocates the standard vaccinations, except in specific cases where there is a medical basis for avoiding them—be writing this foreword? I believe that there is a growing controversy on the subject and Mr. Miller needs to be heard. I need not agree with all of his conclusions in order to recognize a sincere desire to inject new information (and in some cases highlight older information) into the public arena.

Similarly, I see a need for those professionals who are proponents of routine immunizations to explain to a new and perhaps more questioning generation their rationale. They need to respond to Mr. Miller through forums and the media—since the debate is going on less in professional circles than in the popular press as well as on radio and television.

Mr. Miller's book, _Vaccines: Are They Really Safe and Effective?_, is a voice seeking dialogue and requiring counterpoint.

George R. Schwartz, MD
Physician and Toxicologist
Santa Fe, New Mexico

Foreword II

Harold E. Buttram, MD

There is at present time an ominous trend in America towards deteriorating health in children and young adults, a trend which is well substantiated by scientific statistical reports. Allergic diseases such as asthma and eczema are rapidly increasing in both frequency and severity. Autoimmune diseases (afflictions in which antibodies or immune cells attack the tissues of one's own body) have increased manyfold in the past several generations. Perhaps most ominous of all is the rise in childhood behavioral disorders, including hyperactivity and learning disorders, with approximately 15 percent of children now being classified as learning disabled. A substantial portion of today's children are receiving frequent courses of antibiotics for treatment of recurrent ear infections and/or respiratory illness, a pattern which suggests an increasing prevalence of immune impairment when compared with earlier generations. Among young adults of today there are the newly emerging and poorly understood syndromes of chemical sensitivity and chronic fatigue, conditions which are disabling millions of our youth who should be entering the prime of their lives.

Unquestionably there are multiple causes for these adverse health trends. Unhealthful dietary patterns and exposures to toxic environmental chemicals certainly play major roles. However, our concern here is to the possible role that the routine mass inoculation of children may be playing in the increasing patterns of disabled immunity. There is one question which must be addressed: Do vaccination programs stunt or in any way thwart the normal development of the immune systems of children? As admirably reviewed in the present monograph, there are sound grounds for believing that the answer may be in the affirmative. Basing his statements on scientific literature, the author shows that the incidence of many common infections had already been declining as a result of improved sanitation before introduction of vaccines, and that this decline was barely accelerated, if at all, by the vaccines. He also shows that there may be a direct relationship between vaccinations and the modern epidemics of chronic fatigue, autoimmune disorders, AIDS, learning disabilities, and other health problems as well.

In order to better understand the concerns noted above, it would be well to review the development of the immune system following birth. The newborn infant comes into the world with a relatively undeveloped immune system. The infant does carry antibodies from its mother which persist for about six months, but the lymph nodes are small and rudimentary, the plasma cells are sparse in the bone marrow and lymph nodes, and immunoglobulin synthesis is low. Normally, soon after birth, the infant begins to respond to multiple antigenic stimuli from bacterial flora which rapidly populate his skin, upper respiratory tract, and bowel, as well as the microbial and parasitic infections (estimated at one every six weeks) acquired from the environment. This immunologic experience is reflected in progressive hyperplasia of the lymph follicles, a gradual increase in plasma cells, and an increase in immunoglobulin synthesis. In other words, the immature immune system must run a gauntlet of infectious challenges in order to become strong and resistant, a process which under normal circumstances requires 10 to 12 years.

In former times the so-called minor childhood diseases of measles, mumps, and rubella (German measles) may have served a major role in the normal development and strengthening of the immune systems of children. By altering this former pattern with vaccinations, have we set the stage for the serious chronic diseases now occurring with increasing frequency? Once again, has the overall effect been that of stunting the development of the immune systems of children? There are good reasons for believing that this is the case.

The *New York Times* published an article (December 1, 1988) on findings by Dr. John Walker-Smith of St. Bartholomew's Hospital in London, an expert on intestinal diseases of children. In this article Dr. Walker-Smith reported on a sharp increase in Crohn's disease (affecting the small intestines) in children of East Indian origin _who had grown up in Great Britain,_ while in India the disease is "very, very rare indeed." Dr. Walker-Smith believes that the decline of many childhood infections might allow children in the West to grow up without the vigorous development of their immune system defenses that such infections would ordinarily promote.

Additional evidence in support of this hypothesis is found in an earlier report from Afghanistan entitled, "The Adverse Effects of Anti-pyretics in Measles" (_Indian Pediatrics,_ January 1981: 49-52). In this report it was found that those children with measles who were treated with antipyretics, such as aspirin or Tylenol, to lower fever and inhibit the typical skin rash, had significantly prolonged duration of illness and increased incidence of respiratory complications and diarrhea. The remarkable discovery was made that children with the most violent, highly febrile form of the disease and marked skin rash actually had the best prognosis for recovery. Although the authors were cautious in drawing conclusions, it could be inferred that interference with the natural course of the disease significantly dampened the immune responses of the children. If this is true, it may be assumed that the measles vaccine, and possibly others as well, may have a comparable effect.

For these reasons and those reviewed with clarity and thoroughness in the main body of this book, there are grounds for questioning both the safety and efficacy of current childhood vaccination programs. The time is long overdue for a complete reassessment of these procedures. As in all things dealing with human affairs, science thrives best in an atmosphere of freedom. Mandated childhood vaccinations being the antithesis of freedom, the effects of continuing with these programs will be to freeze and crystallize the advances of science in this area. Admittedly, a full review of current procedures will take time, since the legitimate advances of science usually move slowly. In the meantime, as advised by the author, every parent should be allowed full freedom to accept or reject vaccines for their children. They should be allowed the privilege of "informed consent," the same as with any medical procedure that includes the possibility of adverse reactions.

Harold E. Buttram, MD
Family Practice
Quakertown, Pennsylvania

Preface

This book came about as a result of my search to find the truth about vaccines. When my son was born, the matter became important to me. I began by gathering stacks of information from local, state, college, and medical libraries. Much of this information was taken directly from scientific journals. One by one I studied each "mandatory" vaccine. What were the symptoms of the disease it was meant to protect against? If the disease were contracted, how dangerous could it be? I also looked for 1) solid proof that the vaccine was responsible for a general decline in the incidence of the disease, 2) evidence that the vaccine is effective (Does it offer true immunity?), and 3) side effects and safety.

Slowly, the pieces of the puzzle began to fall into place. Many of the vaccines could not show that they were responsible for a decline in the incidence of the disease. Some of the graphs in this book portray this fact by showing how many of these diseases were declining in number and severity on their own, *before* the vaccines were introduced. Many of the vaccines also failed to show evidence of their ability to confer immunity. In fact, some studies show that the disease is more likely to be contracted by those who are vaccinated against it than by those who are left alone. Finally, many of the vaccines are unsafe. Thousands of children have been damaged by them. Seizures, retardation and death are only a few of the many potential "side effects."

In spite of these findings, I was even more shocked to learn that many powerful individuals within the organized medical profession—the Medical-Industrial Complex—including influential members of the World Health Organization (WHO), the American Medical Association (AMA), the American Academy of Pediatrics (AAP), the Centers for Disease Control and Prevention (CDC),the Food and Drug Administration (FDA), major medical journals, hospitals, health professors, scientists, coroners, and the vaccine manufacturers, are aware of much of this information as well, but appear to have an implicit agreement to obscure the facts, minimize the truth, and deceive the public. For years—ever since the early part of this century when the organized medical profession was granted a legal monopoly on health care—it has stifled dissenting individuals within and outside of the profession from making their warnings known. But doctors are merely human; their united front is only a stoic facade that hides their many differences and concerns. For example, some doctors do warn parents about the potential dangers associated with vaccines. A few even require parents to sign a form absolving the doctor from liability if the child is damaged from the shots. Medical experts who refuse to inoculate their own children are also making a powerful statement, as are the medical policymakers who cower to business concerns, or who elect to disregard pertinent data, especially when a whole nation is willing to trust their partial conclusions while placing innocent children into their care.

On the other hand, few parents are prepared to arrive at their own conclusions regarding the vaccine decision. They tenaciously, almost religiously, trust their doctors and pediatricians. They are afraid to ask questions, or to even consider all of their options. Many parents are simply unwilling to take responsibility for health-related decisions. But parents are ultimately responsible for their own health and the health of their children.

I wrote this book so that parents, like yourself, may make more informed decisions regarding vaccines. I do not advocate them, nor do I presume to know what is best for you and your family. I merely try to present the facts in a clear and straightforward manner. Therefore, if after reading this book you still have questions and concerns, I suggest that you study the references in the back of this book, as well as any other pertinent information you can find. In fact, I recommend that you continue with your search for the truth for as long as it takes to arrive at a proper solution to the vaccine dilemma.

Neil Z. Miller
Medical Research Journalist

Childhood Vaccines

Vaccines are injections that contain weakened amounts of the disease germ that they are meant to protect against. They are said to work by stimulating the body to produce antibodies—proteins that defend the body from an invasion by harmful germs. The term "vaccine" is derived from "vacca," the Latin word for cow. This is because the material in cowpox (a disease affecting the udders of cows), was injected into people to protect them against an attack of smallpox.[1]

The idea of vaccinations to prevent disease dates back to 1796. In that year Edward Jenner, a British physician, believed that dairymaids who had caught cowpox (a minor disease), could not catch smallpox (a fatal disease). Jenner then took diseased matter from the hand of Sarah Nelmes, a local dairymaid who had become infected with cowpox, and inserted this matter into the cut arm of James Phipps, a healthy eight-year-old boy. The boy then caught cowpox. Forty-eight days later Jenner inserted smallpox matter into the boy. It had no effect. This was the first recorded vaccination.[2]

Today, several vaccines exist. They are prevalent—even mandatory—in many countries. Most people trust them to be safe and effective. However, findings on several of the more commonly administered vaccines do not support this conclusion.

POLIO

Polio is a contagious disease caused by an intestinal virus that may attack nerve cells of the brain and spinal cord. Symptoms include fever, headache, sore throat, and vomiting. Some victims develop neurological complications, including stiffness of the neck and back, weak muscles, pain in the joints, and paralysis of one or more limbs or respiratory muscles. In severe cases it may be fatal, due to respiratory paralysis.

Treatment consists of putting the patient to bed and allowing the affected limbs to be completely relaxed. If breathing is affected, a respirator may be used. Physical therapy may be required.

13

In 1955, Dr. Jonas Salk, an American physician and scientist, developed a killed-virus (inactivated) vaccine against polio. Shortly thereafter, Dr. Albert Sabin, also an American physician and scientist, developed a live-virus (oral) vaccine against polio. Both vaccines are said to be safe and effective at preventing the disease.

Findings: Many people mistakenly believe that anyone who contracts polio will become paralyzed or die. However, in most infections caused by polio there are few distinctive symptoms.[3] In fact, 95 percent of everyone who is exposed to the natural polio virus won't exhibit any symptoms, even under epidemic conditions.[4,5] About five percent of infected people will experience mild symptoms, such as a sore throat, stiff neck, headache, and fever—often diagnosed as a cold or flu.[6,7] Muscular paralysis has been estimated to occur in about one of every 1,000 people who contract the disease.[8,9] This has lead some scientific researchers to conclude that the small percentage of people who do develop paralytic polio may be anatomically susceptible to the disease. The vast remainder of the population may be naturally immune to the polio germ.[10]

Several studies have shown that _injections_ increase susceptibility to polio. In fact, researchers have known since the early 1900s that paralytic polio often started at the site of an injection.[11,12] When diphtheria and pertussis vaccines were introduced in the 1940s, cases of paralytic polio skyrocketed (Figure 1).[13] This was documented in _Lancet_ and other medical publications.[14-17] For example, in 1995 the _New England Journal of Medicine_ published a study showing that children who received a single injection within one month after receiving a polio vaccine were eight times more likely to contract polio than children who received no injections.[18]

Polio is virtually nonexistent in the United States today. However, according to Dr. Robert Mendelsohn, medical investigator and pediatrician, there is no credible scientific evidence that the vaccine caused polio to disappear.[19] From 1923 to 1953, before the Salk killed-virus vaccine was introduced, the polio death rate in the United States and England had already declined on its own by 47 percent and 55 percent, respectively (Figure 2).[20] Statistics show a similar decline in other European countries as well.[21] And when the vaccine did become available, many European countries questioned its effectiveness and refused to systematically inoculate their citizens. Yet, polio epidemics also ended in these countries.[22]

The number of reported cases of polio _following_ mass inoculations with the killed-virus vaccine was significantly greater

Figure 1:

Polio Cases Skyrocketed After Diphtheria and Pertussis Vaccines were Introduced

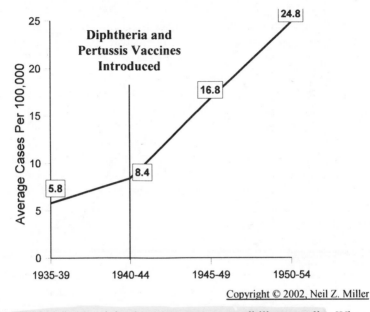

Copyright © 2002, Neil Z. Miller

Several studies show that injections increase susceptibility to polio. When diphtheria and pertussis vaccines were introduced in the 1940s, cases of paralytic poliomyelitis skyrocketed. This chart shows the average number of polio cases per 100,000 people during five year periods before and after the vaccines were introduced. Source: National Morbidity Reports taken from U.S. Public Health surveillance reports; *Lancet* (April 18, 1950), pp. 659-63.

than *before* mass inoculations, and may have more than doubled in the U.S. as a whole. For example, Vermont reported 15 cases of polio during the one-year report period ending August 30, 1954 (before mass inoculations), compared to 55 cases of polio during the one-year period ending August 30, 1955 (after mass inoculations) —a 266% increase. Rhode Island reported 22 cases during the before inoculations period as compared to 122 cases during the after inoculations period—a 454% increase. In New Hampshire the figures were 38-129; in Connecticut they were 144-276; and in Massachusetts they were 273-2027—a whopping 642% increase (Figure 3).[23,24]

Figure 2:

The Polio Death Rate was Decreasing on its Own *Before* the Vaccine was Introduced

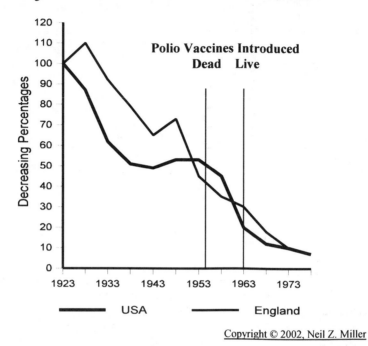

Copyright © 2002, Neil Z. Miller

From 1923 to 1953, before the Salk killed-virus vaccine was introduced, the polio death rate in the United States and England had already declined on its own by 47 percent and 55 percent, respectively. Source: *International Mortality Statistics* (1981) by Michael Alderson.

Doctors and scientists on the staff of the National Institutes of Health during the 1950s were well aware that the Salk vaccine was causing polio. Some frankly stated that it was "worthless as a preventive and dangerous to take."[25] They refused to vaccinate their own children.[26] Health departments banned the inoculations.[27] The Idaho State Health Director angrily declared: "I hold the Salk vaccine and its manufacturers responsible" for a polio outbreak that killed several Idahoans and hospitalized dozens more.[28] Even Salk himself was quoted as saying: "When you inoculate children with a polio vaccine you don't sleep well for two or three weeks."[29] But the National Foundation for Infantile Paralysis, and drug companies

Figure 3:

Cases of Polio *Increased* in the U.S. After Mass Inoculations

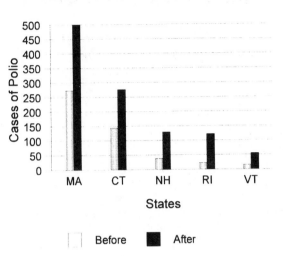

Copyright © 2002, Neil Z. Miller

When national immunization campaigns were initiated in the 1950s, the number of reported cases of polio following mass inoculations with the killed-virus vaccine was significantly greater than before mass inoculations, and may have more than doubled in the U.S. as a whole. Source: U.S. government statistics.

---

with large investments in the vaccine coerced the U.S. Public Health Service into falsely proclaiming the vaccine was safe and effective.[30]

The standards for defining polio were changed when the live-virus polio vaccine was introduced. The new definition of a "polio epidemic" required more cases to be reported. Paralytic polio was redefined as well, making it more difficult to confirm and tally cases. Prior to the introduction of the vaccine the patient only had to exhibit paralytic symptoms for 24 hours. Laboratory confirmation and tests to determine residual (prolonged) paralysis were not required. The new definition required the patient to exhibit paralytic symptoms for at least 60 days, and residual paralysis had to be confirmed twice during the course of the disease. Also, after the vaccine was introduced cases of aseptic meningitis (an infectious disease that is difficult to distinguish from polio) and coxsackie virus infections were reported as separate diseases from polio. But such cases were

Figure 4:

Polio or Aseptic Meningitis?

Sample Months	Reported Cases of Polio	Reported Cases of Aseptic Meningitis
July 1955 (*Before* the new polio definition was introduced)	273	50
July 1961 (*After* the new polio definition was introduced)	65	161
September 1966 (*After* the new polio definition was introduced)	5	256

Copyright © 2002, NZM

Cases of polio were more often reported as aseptic meningitis *after* the vaccine was introduced, skewing efficacy rates. Source: Morbidity and Mortality, Reportable Diseases; *The Los Angeles County Health Index.*

---

counted as polio *before* the vaccine was introduced. Its reported effectiveness was therefore skewed (Figures 4 and 5).[31,32] (The practice of redefining a disease when it supports official immunization goals—despite the questionable ethics—was a common tactic with smallpox as well. For example, in Great Britain the Ministry of Health admitted that the vaccine status of the individual is a guiding factor in diagnosis. In other words, if a person who is vaccinated contracts the disease, the disease is simply recorded under a different name.)[33]

In 1976, Dr. Jonas Salk, creator of the killed-virus vaccine used in the 1950s, testified that the live-virus vaccine (used almost exclusively in the United States from the early 1960s to 2000) was the "principal if not sole cause" of all reported polio cases in the U.S. since 1961.[34] (The virus remains in the throat for one to two weeks and in the feces for up to two months. Thus, vaccine recipients are at risk, and can potentially spread the disease, as long as fecal excretion of the virus continues.)[35] In 1992, the federal Centers for Disease Control and Prevention (CDC) published an admission that the live-virus vaccine had become the dominant cause of polio in the United States.[36] In fact, according to CDC figures, *every case of polio in the U.S. since 1979 was caused by the oral polio vaccine.*[29] Authorities claim the vaccine was responsible for about

Figure 5:

Polio Cases were Predetermined to Decrease when the Medical Definition of Polio was Changed

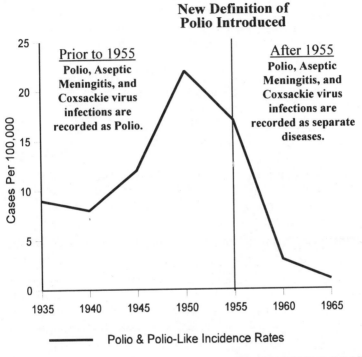

New Definition of Polio Introduced

Prior to 1955
Polio, Aseptic Meningitis, and Coxsackie virus infections are recorded as Polio.

After 1955
Polio, Aseptic Meningitis, and Coxsackie virus infections are recorded as separate diseases.

Cases Per 100,000

——— Polio & Polio-Like Incidence Rates

Copyright © 2002, Neil Z. Miller

Source: *Congressional Hearings,* May 1962; National Morbidity Reports taken from U.S. Public Health surveillance reports.

---

eight cases of polio every year.[38] However, an independent study that analyzed the government's own vaccine database during a recent period of less than five years uncovered 13,641 reports of adverse events following use of the oral polio vaccine. These reports included 6,364 emergency room visits and 540 deaths.[39,40] Public outrage at these tragedies became the impetus for removing the oral polio vaccine from immunization schedules.[41-43]

Fact sheets on polio, published by the U.S. Department of Health and Human Services, warn parents that the inactivated polio vaccine

(IPV) can cause "serious problems *or even death...*"[44] The vaccine maker warns that Guillain-Barré syndrome, a debilitating ailment characterized by muscular incapacitation and nervous system damage, "has been temporally related to administration of another inactivated poliovirus vaccine."[45] And although this company makes the claim that "no causal relationship has been established," it also admits that "deaths have occurred" after vaccination of infants with IPV.[46] Yet, like the days of old, despite these "danger alerts," medical authorities continue to assure parents that the currently available inactivated polio vaccine is both safe and effective.

Polio Vaccines and Cancer: In 1959, Bernice Eddy discovered that polio vaccines being administered throughout the world contained an infectious agent capable of causing cancer.[47,48] In 1960, Drs. Ben Sweet and M.R. Hilleman, of the Merck Institute for Therapeutic Research, were credited with discovering this infectious agent—SV-40, a simian virus that infected nearly all of the monkeys whose kidneys were used to produce polio vaccines. Hilleman and Sweet found SV-40 in all three types of Albert Sabin's live oral polio vaccine, and noted the possibility that it might cause cancer, "especially when administered to human babies."[49,50]

Further research into SV-40 uncovered even more disturbing information. This cancer-causing virus was not only ingested via Sabin's contaminated oral sugar-cube vaccine, but was directly injected into people's bloodstreams as well. Apparently, SV-40 survived the formaldehyde Salk used to kill microbes that defiled his injectable vaccine.[51,52] Experts estimate that between 1954 and 1963, 30 million to 100 million Americans and perhaps another 100 million or more people throughout the world were exposed to SV-40 through ill-conceived polio eradication campaigns (Figure 6).[53,54]

Studies in eminent journals throughout the world appear to confirm that SV-40 is a catalyst for many types of cancer.[55-74] It has been found in brain tumors and leukemia.[75] In 1996, Michele Carbone, a molecular pathologist at Chicago's Loyola University Medical Center, was able to detect SV-40 in 38 percent of patients with bone cancer and in 58 percent of those with mesothelioma, a deadly type of lung cancer.[76-78] Carbone's research indicates that SV-40 blocks an important protein that normally protects cells from becoming malignant.[79] In 1998, a national cancer database was analyzed: 17 percent more bone cancers, 20 percent more brain cancers, and 178 percent more mesotheliomas were found in people who were exposed to SV-40-tainted polio vaccines.[80]

<u>**Figure 6:**</u>

Polio Vaccines and Simian Virus #40

**1. Monkey kidneys are used
to develop polio vaccines.**

**2. SV-40, a cancer-causing
virus, thrived in monkey kidneys.**

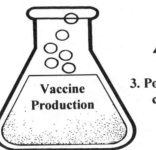

Vaccine
Production

**3. Polio vaccines were
contaminated.**

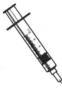

**4. Millions of people in the USA
and throughout the world
were infected.**

**5. Cancer rates have increased.
SV-40 is found in brain tumors, bone
cancers, lung cancers, and leukemia.**

<u>Copyright © 2002, Neil Z. Miller</u>

Perhaps the most alarming aspect of this ongoing simian virus debacle can be found in other studies suggesting that SV-40, introduced to humans through the polio vaccine, can be passed from human to human and from mother to child. A study of nearly 59,000 women found that children of mothers who received the Salk vaccine between 1959 and 1965 had brain tumors at a rate 13 times greater than mothers who did not receive those polio shots.[81-83]

Another study published in the U.S. medical journal *Cancer Research* found SV-40 present in 23 percent of blood samples and 45 percent of semen taken from healthy subjects.[84,85] Apparently, the virus is being spread sexually and from mother to child in the womb. According to biology and genetics professor Mauro Tognon, one of the study's authors, this would explain why brain, bone, and lung cancers are on the rise—a 30 percent increase in U.S. brain tumors alone over the past 25 years—and why SV-40 was detected in brain tumors of children born after 1965 who presumably did not receive polio vaccines containing the virus.[86,87]

Despite official denials of any correlation between polio vaccines, SV-40 and increased cancer rates,[88] by April 2001, 62 papers from 30 laboratories around the world had reported SV-40 in human tissues and tumors.[89] The virus was also discovered in pituitary and thyroid tumors, and in patients with kidney disease.[90]

Polio Vaccines and AIDS: SV-40, the cancer-causing monkey virus found in polio vaccines and administered to millions of unsuspecting people throughout the world, was just one of _numerous_ simian viruses known to have contaminated polio vaccines.[91-93] "As monkey kidney culture is host to innumerable simian viruses, the number found varying in relation to the amount of work expended to find them, the problem presented to the manufacturer is considerable, if not insuperable," one early vaccine researcher wrote to a congressional panel studying the safety of growing live polio-virus vaccine in monkey kidneys.[94] "As our technical methods improve we may find fewer and fewer lots of vaccine which can be called free from simian virus."[95]

According to Harvard Medical School professor Ronald Desrosier, the practice of growing polio vaccines in monkey kidneys is "a ticking time bomb."[96] Evidently, some viruses can live inside monkeys without causing harm. But if these viruses were to somehow cross species and enter the human population, new diseases could occur. Desrosier continued: "The danger in using monkey tissue to produce human vaccines is that some viruses produced by monkeys may be transferred to humans in the vaccine, with very bad health consequences."[97] Desrosier also warned that testing can only be done for _known_ viruses, and that our knowledge is limited to about "two percent of existing monkey viruses."[98]

Virus detection techniques were crude and unreliable during the 1950s, 60s, and 70s when polio vaccines were initially produced and dispensed. It wasn't until the mid 1980s that new and more sophisticated testing procedures were developed.[99,100] That was when researchers discovered that about 50 percent of all African green monkeys—the primate of choice for making polio vaccines—were infected with simian immunodeficiency virus (SIV), a virus closely related to human immunodeficiency virus (HIV), the infectious agent thought to precede AIDS.[101-104] This caused some researchers to wonder whether HIVs may simply be SIVs "residing in and adapting to a human host."[105] It caused others to suspect that SIV may have mutated into HIV once it was introduced into the human population by way of contaminated polio vaccines.[106-110] In fact, according to Robert Gallo, an expert on the AIDS virus, some versions of the SIV monkey virus are virtually indistinguishable from some human variants of HIV: "The monkey virus *is* the human virus. There are monkey viruses as close to isolates of HIV-2 as HIV-2 isolates are to each other."[111]

Today's Vaccine: Despite the polio vaccine's long history of animal-virus contamination, today's inactivated shot is manufactured in much the same way as earlier versions: "The viruses are grown in cultures of a continuous line of monkey kidney cells...supplemented with newborn calf serum..." The vaccine also contains two antibiotics (neomycin and streptomycin) plus formaldehyde.[112] In Canada, the inactivated polio vaccine is produced in human fetal tissue.[113] In other parts of the world, new highly virulent strains of polio—caused by mutations and "recombinations" within the *oral* polio vaccine—are inducing unprecedented outbreaks of paralysis and death.[114-117]

TETANUS

Tetanus is a non-contagious bacterial disease that causes severe muscular contractions. It is also called *lockjaw* because some victims are unable to open their mouths or swallow. Other symptoms include depression, headaches, and spasms that interfere with breathing.[118,119]

Tetanus is caused by toxins produced by a bacterium called *Clostridium tetani*. The dormant germs (spores) live in soil, dust, and manure. They can enter the body through cuts and puncture wounds, but will only multiply in an anaerobic (oxygen-free) environment. The incubation period, from the time of the injury until the first symptoms appear, ranges from a few days to three weeks. However, careful attention to wound hygiene will eliminate the possibility of tetanus in most cases. Deep puncture wounds and wounds with a lot of dead tissue should be thoroughly cleaned and not allowed to close until healing has occurred beneath the skin.[120]

A *tetanus toxoid vaccine* became available in 1933. A *tetanus immune globulin* (TIG) injection—an antitoxin—is also available.

This shot may be administered to persons with low tetanus antibody levels (including unvaccinated individuals) shortly after a serious wound occurs. This injection introduces tetanus-fighting antibodies directly into the body. The antibody levels achieved with TIG are often adequate to defend against the disease.[121,122]

Findings: During the mid-1800s, there were 205 cases of tetanus per 100,000 wounds among U.S. military personnel. By the early 1900s, this rate had declined to 16 cases per 100,000 wounds —a 92 percent reduction. During the mid-1940s, the incidence of tetanus dropped even further to .44 cases per 100,000 wounds.[123] Some researchers attribute this decline to an increased attention to wound hygiene.[124,125]

Today, authorities claim that tetanus infects about 500,000 people each year worldwide, primarily in developing countries.[126] However, in the United States, from 1990 to 1999 (a 10-year period), there were a total of 473 cases of tetanus—an average of 47 cases per year. Of these, 70 died—about seven people per year. The case-fatality rate was 15 percent (Figure 7).[127] In Australia, there are about 10 cases of tetanus per year with a case-fatality rate of 10 percent.[128] In Canada, there have been about five cases of tetanus annually in recent years, with no deaths recorded since 1991.[129]

During the 1970s and 1980s, approximately 70 percent of all cases of tetanus in the United States, and 80 percent of all cases in Australia, occurred in adults over the age of 50 years.[130-133] About 95 percent of all tetanus fatalities occurred in this age group. Only five percent of tetanus cases in the U.S. were in persons less than 20 years of age, and these were rarely fatal.[134]

During the 1990s, the percentage of cases among persons aged 25-59 years increased. For example, in 1999 there were 40 cases of tetanus. Five cases (12.5 percent) were in persons younger than 25 years; 13 cases (32.5 percent) were in persons older than 59 years; 22 cases (55 percent) were among persons aged 25-59 years. Seven of the 22 cases in this age group occurred in intravenous drug users; two of these cases were fatal.[135]

Numerous studies and case reports have linked the tetanus vaccine to severe and even fatal reactions, including neurological and paralytic disorders such as Guillain-Barré syndrome (GBS), demyelinating diseases, arthritis, joint inflammation, anaphylactic shock, and other life-threatening allergic reactions.[136-161]

The *New England Journal of Medicine* published a study showing that tetanus booster vaccinations cause T-lymphocyte blood

Figure 7:

Tetanus Cases and Deaths: United States, 1990-1999

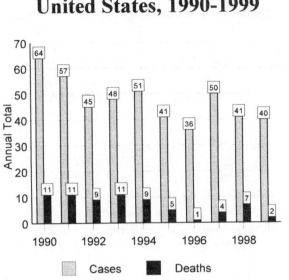

In the United States, from 1990 to 1999 (a 10-year period), there were a total of 473 cases of tetanus—an average of 47 cases per year. Of these, 70 died—about seven people per year. The case-fatality rate was 15 percent. Source: CDC. *MMWR* 1999; 48(No. 53):84-90.

count ratios to drop below normal. The greatest decrease occurred up to two weeks later. The authors of the study noted that these altered ratios are similar to those found in victims of HIV/AIDS.[162] Even a brief suppression of normal T-lymphocyte ratios is undesirable, and may be the underlying cause of at least one immunological disorder found in infants.[163]

In 1994, The U.S. Institute of Medicine (IOM) corroborated a causal relationship between tetanus toxoid, brachial neuritis, and Guillain-Barré syndrome.[164] The IOM also reported on several cases of anaphylactic reactions—severe, life-threatening allergic responses resulting in swelling of the mouth, inability to breathe, shock, collapse, or death—within four hours of tetanus vaccine injections.[165]

In 1997, *Epidemiology* published a study comparing asthma and allergy rates in unvaccinated children versus children who received a vaccine containing tetanus. None of the unvaccinated children had recorded asthma episodes or consultations for asthma or other allergic illnesses before age 10 years. In the vaccinated children, 23 percent had asthma episodes and asthma consultations, while 30 percent had consultations for other allergic illnesses. Similar differences were observed at 5 and 16 years of age.[166]

In 2000, a new study in the _Journal of Manipulative and Physiological Therapeutics_ confirmed earlier findings that children who receive DPT or tetanus vaccines are significantly more likely to develop a "history of asthma" or other "allergy-related respiratory symptoms" than those who remain unvaccinated. The study was conducted from 1988 to 1994 and included data from nearly 14,000 infants, children, and adolescents, aged two months to 16 years. A child who received the DPT or tetanus vaccination was 50 percent more likely to experience severe allergic reactions, 80 percent more likely to experience sinusitis, and twice as likely to develop asthma. In fact, the authors of the study calculated that "Fifty percent of diagnosed asthma cases (2.93 million) in U.S. children and adolescents would be prevented if the DPT or tetanus vaccination was not administered. Similarly, 45 percent of sinusitis cases (4.94 million) and 54 percent of allergy-related episodes of nose and eye symptoms (10.54 million) in a 12-month period would be prevented after discontinuation of the vaccine."[167]

MEASLES

Measles is a contagious disease caused by a virus that affects the respiratory system, skin, and eyes. Symptoms include a high fever, cough, runny nose, sore, red and sensitive eyes. Small pink spots with gray-white centers develop inside the mouth. Itchy pink spots break out on the face and spread over the body. Symptoms usually disappear after one to two weeks. Treatment mainly consists of allowing the disease to run its course.

Prior to the 1960s, most children in the United States and Canada caught measles. Complications from the disease were unlikely. Previously healthy children usually recovered without incident.[168] However, measles can be dangerous in populations newly exposed to the virus,[169] and in malnourished children living in undeveloped countries.[170,171] In advanced countries, measles can be severe when it infects people living in impoverished communities with poor nutrition, sanitation, and inadequate health care.[172] Complications are also more likely when the disease strikes infants, adults, and anyone with a compromised immune system.[173] (Several studies show that when patients with measles are given vitamin A supplements, their complication rates and chances of dying are significantly reduced.)[174-179]

Doctors and other health authorities often try to frighten parents by exaggerating the risks. For example, vaccine pamphlets published by the CDC claim that 1 out of every 1000 children who contract measles will get encephalitis, an infection of the brain.[180] However, Dr. Robert Mendelsohn, renowned pediatrician and vaccine researcher, had this to say: "The incidence of 1/1000 may be accurate for children who live in conditions of poverty and malnutrition" but for just about everyone else "the incidence of true encephalitis is probably more like 1/10,000 or 1/100,000."[181] Furthermore, about 75 percent of these cases will *not* show evidence of brain damage.[182]

Before the 1960s, most children in the U.S. caught measles. In 1963, a team of scientists, headed by American researcher John Enders, created a measles vaccine. Mass inoculations soon followed.

Findings: A significant decline in measles began long before the vaccine was introduced. From 1958 to 1962, the number of cases toppled by 38 percent.[183] The death rate tumbled on its own even more. In 1900, there were 13.3 measles deaths in the United States per 100,000 population. By 1955, eight years *before* the first measles shot, the death rate had declined on its own by 97.7 percent to .03 deaths per 100,000.[184] Figures published in *International Mortality Statistics* confirm this reduction: from 1915 to 1958, the measles death rate in the U.S. and U.K. declined by 98 percent (Figure 8).[185]

The measles vaccine does not confer permanent immunity. Epidemics regularly occur in vaccinated populations. Dr. William Atkinson, senior epidemiologist with the CDC, admitted that "measles transmission has been clearly documented among vaccinated persons. In some large outbreaks...over 95 percent of cases have a history of vaccination."[186] In fact, according to the World Health Organization (WHO), the chances are about 15 times greater that measles will be contracted by those vaccinated against the disease than by those who are left alone.[187]

The medical literature is replete with documented vaccine failures. For example, In 1988, 69 percent of all school-aged children in the U.S. who contracted measles were vaccinated.[188] In 1989, 89 percent of all school-aged measles victims in the U.S. had been vaccinated.[189] In 1995, 56 percent of all measles cases in the U.S. occurred in people who were previously vaccinated (Figure 9).[190]

Figure 8:

The Measles Death Rate was Decreasing on its Own *Before* the Vaccine was Introduced

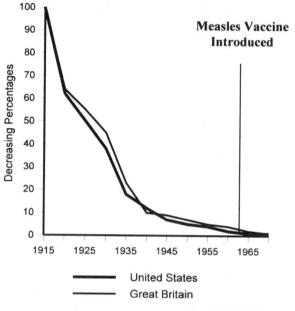

Copyright © 2002, Neil Z. Miller

From 1915 to 1958, before the measles vaccine was introduced, the measles death rate in the United States and Great Britain had already declined on its own by 98 percent. Source: *International Mortality Statistics,* 1981.

In 1996, this pattern persisted: measles outbreaks occurred primarily among children who had prior vaccinations.[191] And in 1999, the CDC continued to document numerous cases of measles in previously vaccinated individuals.[192]

The measles vaccine has a long history of causing serious adverse reactions. The pharmaceutical company responsible for producing the measles vaccine publishes an extensive list of ailments known to have occurred following the shot. Severe afflictions affecting nearly every body system—blood, lymphatic, digestive, cardiovascular, immune, nervous, respiratory, and sensory—have been linked to this "preventive" inoculation. These include: encephalitis, subacute

Figure 9:

Outbreaks of Measles
in Vaccinated Populations

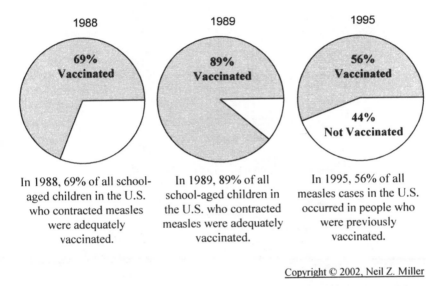

Copyright © 2002, Neil Z. Miller

Source: *Infect Med* 1997; 14(4):297-300, 310. Several CDC *Morbidity and Mortality Weekly Reports.*

---

sclerosing panencephalitis, Guillain-Barré syndrome, febrile and afebrile convulsions, seizures, ataxia, ocular palsies, anaphylaxis, angioneurotic edema, bronchial spasms, panniculitis, vasculitis, atypical measles, thrombocytopenia, lymphadenopathy, leukocytosis, pneumonitis, Stevens-Johnson syndrome, erythema multiforme, urticaria, deafness, otitis media, retinitis, optic neuritis, rash, fever, dizziness, headache, and death.[193] A recent study in *Lancet* found a link between this vaccine and bowel disease. People who received the measles vaccine were 2½ times more likely to develop ulcerative colitis and three times more likely to develop Crohn's disease when compared to unvaccinated controls (Figure 10).[194]

The measles vaccine dramatically altered distribution of the disease by shifting incidence rates from age-groups unlikely to experience problems (children 5 to 9 years old) to age-groups most likely to suffer from severe complications (infants, teenagers, and

Figure 10:

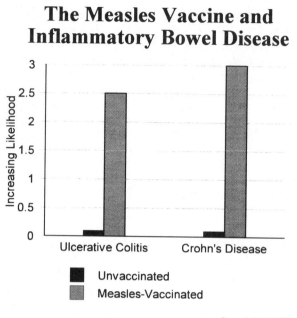

The Measles Vaccine and Inflammatory Bowel Disease

Copyright © 2002, Neil Z. Miller

People who received the measles vaccine were 2½ times more likely to develop ulcerative colitis and three times more likely to develop Crohn's disease when compared to unvaccinated controls. Source: _Lancet_ 1995; 345: 1071-1074.

---

adults). Before the vaccine was introduced, it was extremely rare for an infant to contract measles. However, by the 1990s more than 25 percent of all measles cases were occurring in babies under a year of age. CDC officials admit this situation is likely to get worse, and attribute it to the growing number of mothers who were vaccinated during the 1960s, 1970s, and 1980s. (When natural immunity is denied, moms can no longer pass protective maternal antibodies to their babies.)[195] In 1999, _Pediatrics_ confirmed that infants of mothers born after 1963 are 7½ times more likely to contract the disease than infants of mothers born earlier.[196]

The risk of measles-related pneumonia and liver abnormalities is greater in adolescent and young adult age-groups. According to a study in the _Journal of Infectious Diseases,_ such complications have increased by as much as 20 percent.[197] The risk of death from measles is also much higher for infants and adults than for children.[198]

The following excerpt is from a statement made by a mother testifying before Congress (*Hearing Before the Subcommittee on Health and the Environment*) regarding vaccine injury compensation:

"My name is Wendy Scholl. I reside in the state of Florida with my husband, Gary, and three daughters, Stacy, Holly, and Jackie. Let me stress that all three of our daughters were born healthy, normal babies. I am here to tell of Stacy's reaction to the measles vaccine...where according to the medical profession, anything within 7 to 10 days after the vaccine to do with neurological sequelae or seizures or brain damage fits a measles reaction...

"At 16 months old, Stacy received her measles shot. She was a happy, healthy, normal baby, typical, curious, playful until the 10th day after her shot when I walked into her room to find her laying in her crib, flat on her stomach, her head twisted to one side. Her eyes were glassy and affixed.

"She was panting, struggling to breathe. Her small head lay in a pool of blood that hung from her mouth. It was a terrifying sight, yet at that point I didn't realize that my happy, bouncing baby was never to be the same again.

"When we arrived at the emergency room, Stacy's temperature was 107 degrees. The first four days of Stacy's hospital stay she battled for life. She was in a coma and had kidney failure. Her lungs filled with fluid and she had ongoing seizures.

"Her diagnosis was 'post-vaccinal encephalitis' and her prognosis was grave. She was paralyzed on her left side, prone to seizures, had visual problems. However, we were told by doctors we were extremely lucky. I didn't feel lucky.

"We were horrified that this vaccine which was given only to ensure that she would have a safer childhood, almost killed her. I didn't know that the possibility of this type of reaction even existed. But now, it is our reality."[199]

MUMPS

Mumps is a contagious disease caused by a virus. The illness begins with a fever, headache, muscle aches, and fatigue. Salivary glands beneath the ears along the jaw line become swollen. In some instances, testicles, ovaries, and female breasts may also swell.

Treatment mainly consists of allowing the disease to run its course. Medical intervention is seldom required. Symptoms usually disappear within a week. The disease confers permanent immunity; the infected person will not contract it again.[200,201]

Findings: Mumps is a relatively harmless disease when it is experienced in childhood.[202] Complications are uncommon but can be much more severe when they occur in teenagers and adults.[203-205] For example, orchitis (inflammation of the testes) occurs in about 20 percent of mumps cases in post-pubescent males.[206] This has caused some authorities to claim mumps will prevent a man from fathering children. However, orchitis usually affects only one testicle; sterility from the ailment is extremely rare.[207,208]

Mumps has also been associated with transient meningitis, temporary hearing loss, and inflammation of the ovaries.[209] Full recovery without complications usually follows in a few days.[210] Permanent sequelae, including deaths from mumps, are very rare.[211] For example, one mumps-related death was reported in 1991.[212]

During the early 1980s, there were about 4000 cases per year.[213] In 1995, there were less than 1000 documented cases in the U.S.[214] However, artificial immunity conferred by the mumps vaccine does not last. Studies show substantial numbers of cases of mumps among persons previously vaccinated against the disease. For example, in 1987 there was an outbreak of mumps in Minnesota schools; 632 of the 769 cases (82 percent) were in previously vaccinated students.[215] That same year, 119 stockbrokers at the Chicago futures stock exchange contracted mumps "following an intensified push for mumps vaccination."[216,217] And in 1991, there was an outbreak of mumps in Tennessee schools; 67 of the 68 cases (99 percent) were in previously vaccinated students.[218]

Prior to the introduction of the mumps vaccine, most children under 10 years of age contracted mumps.[219] However, the mumps vaccine shifted incidence rates from young children to teenagers and adults. Mumps in young children is a mild, benign disease. It is a more serious disease when contracted by older age groups.[220]

From 1967 to 1971, before the mumps vaccine was put into general use, 92 percent of all cases occurred in persons 14 years of age or younger. Just eight percent of cases occurred in teenagers 15 years of age or older.[221] By 1987, several years after the vaccine was being administered on a national scale, 38 percent of all cases were occurring in this older age group.[222]

The drug company that produces the mumps vaccine publishes an extensive list of ailments known to have occurred following the mumps or MMR (measles, mumps, and rubella) shot. These include aseptic meningitis, encephalitis, orchitis, diabetes mellitus, parotitis (the technical name for mumps), anaphylaxis, and death.[223]

In 1986, researchers published data on several children who

developed diabetes 2 to 4 weeks after mumps vaccination.[224] By 1990, several new cases of diabetes within 30 days following vaccination were reported.[225] In 1991, scientists reported a case of Type-1 diabetes occurring five months following mumps vaccination.[226] That same year, other researchers documented several cases of diabetes and pancreatitis after mumps vaccination.[227] In 1992, 180 European doctors jointly noted that the mumps vaccine "can trigger diabetes, which only becomes apparent months after vaccination."[228] That same year, the *New England Journal of Medicine* published data confirming that viruses are capable of triggering diabetes.[229] Today, the U.S. government continues to receive reports of diabetes following receipt of the MMR vaccine.[230]

In 1993, *Lancet* published data confirming aseptic meningitis as a well-recognized complication of mumps vaccine, with onset typically occurring 15 to 35 days after receiving the shot.[231] That same year, Japan removed the MMR vaccine from the market because it was causing encephalitis in 1 of every 1044 people vaccinated.[232] And in 1994, the U.S. Institute of Medicine acknowledged being able to isolate and identify the mumps vaccine-virus strain from neurologically impaired patients following vaccination. Aseptic meningitis was officially recognized as resulting from the mumps vaccine.[233]

RUBELLA

Rubella (or German Measles) is a contagious disease caused by a virus. Symptoms include a slight fever, rash, sore throat and runny nose. Lymph nodes on the back of the head, behind the ears, and on the side of the neck may become tender. In some instances, the joints may become painful and swollen.

Treatment mainly consists of allowing the disease to run its course. Medical intervention is seldom required. Symptoms usually disappear within a few days. Most cases confer permanent immunity; rubella rarely infects the same person twice.[234]

Findings: Rubella is essentially a tame disease when contracted by children. The illness is usually so mild it escapes detection or passes for a cold. However, if a pregnant woman develops the disease during the first trimester, her baby may be born with birth defects.[235]

In 1969, the first live rubella virus vaccine was licensed in the United States. Several European countries, Canada, and Japan also introduced rubella vaccines around this time. In 1979, vaccine manufacturers started producing and distributing the Wistar RA27/3 strain of the live rubella virus "adapted to and propagated in WI-38 human diploid lung fibroblasts."[236] In common language, this vaccine originated from cell lines obtained from the tissue of aborted fetuses.[237-241] This vaccine is still in use today.

The drug company that produces the rubella vaccine publishes an extensive list of ailments known to have occurred following the rubella (or MMR) shot. These include arthritis, arthralgia, myalgia, Guillain-Barré syndrome, polyneuritis, polyneuropathy, anaphylaxis, and death.[242] Several studies have documented these and other afflictions following rubella vaccination. For example, separate studies in *Lancet* and the *Journal of Infectious Diseases* documented "rubella-associated arthritis" and chronic arthritis in women following their rubella shots.[243-245] Another study in *Annals of the Rheumatic Diseases* showed that 55 percent of women vaccinated against rubella developed arthritis or joint pain within four weeks (Figure 11).[246]

Several researchers have documented correlations between the rubella vaccine and neurological disorders.[247-252] Others have found a connection to diabetes.[253-256] Additional studies have linked the rubella vaccine to Chronic Fatigue syndrome, a debilitating immune system disorder.[257,258] According to the author of one study, "In countries that routinely immunize children with the new [rubella] vaccine, adults might be persistently reexposed to the more provocative antigens of the new vaccine due to respiratory secretions..."[259] In other words, the rubella virus lingers in recently vaccinated children and can be spread to hypersensitive adults. Reinfection produces multiple viral antibodies resulting in "the characteristic symptoms in adult women who are over-represented in the patient population."[260] Thus, "the possible role of rubella immunization in the etiology of chronic fatigue syndromes deserves further study."[261]

The following excerpts typify the adverse possibilities:

"I am a nursing student. Within three weeks of taking the MMR vaccine I began feeling weak, tired, and sluggish. This lead to numbness in both hands and feet. I developed Guillain-Barré syndrome and was hospitalized for two months. I was unable to walk, had difficulty moving my upper extremities, suffered urinary and abdominal problems, partial facial paralysis, and I lost a substantial amount of weight. Previously, I was an active, healthy woman. My doctors do not know how I developed this syndrome."

"My child caught rubella two weeks after her MMR."

"After the birth of my daughter, my obstetrician recommended

Figure 11:

The Rubella Vaccine and Arthritis

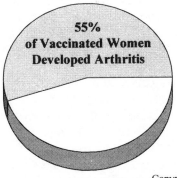

55%
of Vaccinated Women
Developed Arthritis

Copyright © 2002, Neil Z. Miller

In a study of adult women who were vaccinated against rubella, 55 percent developed arthritis or joint pain within four weeks. Source: *Annals of the Rheumatic Diseases* 1986; 45:110-114.

---

the MMR vaccine since I didn't have antibodies. A week after the shot, a rash appeared all over my body. Two weeks later, I had severe joint pain which alternated from my knee to ankle to wrist. The joint pain lasted seven days, and then severe fatigue set in. My doctor immediately said this was not related to the vaccine."

"I am a 57-year-old registered nurse who was, as a condition of employment, required to take an MMR. About 14 days later I developed a rash with lesions in my right eye, fever, and joint pain. My joint pain has not gone away but has become chronic, and sometimes unbearable. I have been put on a variety of drugs, which I have had terrible reactions to, and was even hospitalized for. I have been unable to work. I did file a worker's compensation claim, which they are trying to deny."[262]

Prior to the introduction of the rubella vaccine in 1969, thousands of cases of rubella circulated throughout society. Most children contracted the disease and developed permanent protection. As a result, about 85 percent of the adult population was naturally immune.[263-265] After the vaccine was introduced, researchers began to notice that cases of the disease were occurring in vaccinated populations. In fact, serological surveys have confirmed that about

15 percent of the adult population, including women of childbearing age, are still not protected from the disease—the same percentage as before vaccinations.[266-268]

From 1966 to 1968, *before* the rubella vaccine was licensed, 77 percent of all cases occurred in persons 14 years of age or younger. Just 23 percent of all cases occurred in persons 15 years of age or older.[269] By 1990, however, 81 percent of all rubella cases were in the 15-or-older group, with the greatest increases in persons 15 to 29 years old—the prime childbearing years.[270] From 1994 to 1997 this trend continued, with 85 percent of all rubella cases occurring in persons 15 years or older.[271]

Since 1969, when the rubella vaccine was introduced, the number of rubella cases has steadily declined. For example, in 1970 more than 56,000 cases were recorded in the United States; 3,904 in 1980; 1,125 in 1990; just 152 in 2000.[272-273] Authorities use this as evidence of the vaccine's efficacy and benefit to society. However, the vaccine's capacity to reduce the number of rubella cases is inconsequential if it is unable to protect the unborn child from birth defects.[274] In fact, when the data is analyzed, it becomes clear that just the opposite is true. Misguided vaccine strategies that shifted rubella cases to more risky age groups apparently caused an *increase* in congenital rubella syndrome (CRS) related birth defects.[275]

In 1966, the year the government began keeping statistics on congenital rubella syndrome, there were 11 cases reported in the United States. In 1967, there were just 10 cases, with 14 more reported the following year. However, in 1969 the rubella vaccine was introduced and the CDC recorded 31 cases of CRS. In 1970, CRS cases skyrocketed to 77—a greater than 600 percent increase over pre-vaccine numbers. In 1971, there were 68 cases. These figures remained high in subsequent years (Figure 12).[276] Adjustments for annual population variances do not alter the results.[277] By 1991, there were just 1,401 cases of rubella, but the CDC recorded 47 cases of CRS. In 1992, rubella cases dropped to 160, and there were just 11 cases of CRS—the exact number recorded by the CDC more than 25 years earlier in 1966 *before* the vaccine was introduced.[278]

The *New England Journal of Medicine* reported that one-third of all hospital employees rejected rubella shots; 81 percent of the doctors refused the vaccine, with senior staff physicians having an even lower participation rate.[279] Shortly thereafter, the *Journal of the American Medical Association* reported that 47 percent of all employees at the University of Southern California Medical Center would not comply with a rubella vaccination campaign; 78 percent

Figure 12:

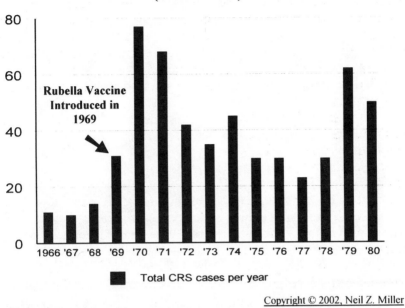

Congenital Rubella Syndrome
(Total Cases)

Rubella Vaccine
Introduced in
1969

Total CRS cases per year

Copyright © 2002, Neil Z. Miller

Cases of congenital rubella syndrome (CRS) *increased* after the rubella vaccine was introduced. Source: CDC. *MMWR* (October 25, 1996).

---

of the doctors would not consent to the shots, while 91 percent of the obstetricians and gynecologists (who work daily with pregnant women) refused to participate (Figure 13).[280,281] Such reluctance on the part of physicians prompted Dr. Robert Mendelsohn to pose the following ethical question: "If doctors themselves are afraid of the vaccine, why on earth should the law require that you and other parents allow them to administer it to your kids?"[282]

DIPHTHERIA

Diphtheria is a contagious bacterial disease of the upper respiratory system. It is mainly spread by the coughing and sneezing of infected persons. The first symptoms appear two to five days after infection. They include a sore throat, headache, coughing, fever, and swollen lymph nodes in the neck. As the disease progresses,

Figure 13:

Doctors Refuse the Rubella Vaccine

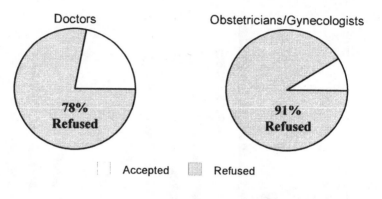

Copyright © 2002, Neil Z. Miller

In one study, 78 percent of the doctors and 91 percent of the obstetricians and gynecologists (who work daily with pregnant women) refused to take a rubella shot. Source: _Journal of the American Medical Association_; 245(7):711-13.

---

a thick membrane forms on the surface of the tonsils and throat, and may extend into the windpipe and lungs. This membrane may interfere with breathing and swallowing. In severe cases, it can completely block the breathing passages and cause death if not treated. Other complications include inflammation of the heart muscle and respiratory paralysis.[283]

Diphtheria requires medical attention but is treatable with common antibiotics such as penicillin. Heart failure is treated with medication, while a respirator is used to aid in breathing.[284] A diphtheria antitoxin became available in 1895 and is still used today. It can be administered to persons with low diphtheria antibody levels or immediately after being exposed to the disease.[285] A diphtheria vaccine was introduced in the 1920s. Widespread use of this modified toxoid began in the 1940s when it was combined with the tetanus and pertussis vaccines (DPT).[286,287]

Findings: Diphtheria was a common disease during the late 19th century. For example, from 1891 to 1895, New York averaged 7,200 cases per year.[288,289] The case-fatality rate was about five percent.[290,291] In the U.S. during the 1940s, the number of diphtheria cases fluctuated between 15,000 and 30,000 annually.[292] However, in 1980 a new pattern emerged, with only a few cases each year.[293] From 1990 to 2000 (an 11-year period), 25 cases of diphtheria were recorded. Three of these cases were fatal.[294,295]

The diphtheria death rate plummeted long before the vaccine was introduced. In the United States, from 1900 to 1930, diphtheria fatalities declined by more than 85 percent.[296] In fact, mortality from the disease decreased from 7.2 deaths per 10,000 in 1911 to .9 deaths per 10,000 in 1935—an 88 percent decline.[297]

In 1975, the Food and Drug Administration (FDA) concluded that diphtheria toxoid "is not as effective an immunizing agent as might be anticipated." Authorities confessed that diphtheria may occur in vaccinated individuals, and noted that "the permanence of immunity induced by the toxoid...is open to question.[298]

In 1979, authorities changed the medical definition of diphtheria. Prior to the change, "cutaneous" and "inhalation" cases of the disease were counted. After the change, only inhalation cases were labeled as bona fide diphtheria. As a result, official statistics showed an immediate 95 percent decline in cases the following year (and a 99.3 percent reduction from 1970 to 1980). The number of diphtheria cases remained low every year thereafter.[299]

During the mid-1990s, there were outbreaks of diphtheria in eastern Europe and the newly independent states of the former Soviet Union. Many of the cases occurred in persons who were properly vaccinated. As a result, authorities questioned the merits of diphtheria vaccination programs.[300,301]

In 1999, FDA announced that diphtheria vaccines given to children during the previous year were "too weak to protect against diphtheria."[302] However, since diphtheria is very rare in the United States and other developed countries, officials did not recommend new vaccines for children who received the worthless ones.[303]

PERTUSSIS

Pertussis is a contagious disease caused by a bacterium that affects the respiratory system. Sometimes called whooping cough, this disease got its name from the high-pitched whooping noise victims make when they try to catch their breath after severe coughing attacks. Symptoms progress through three stages. In the first stage, which usually lasts one to two weeks, victims have trouble breathing, and may develop a cough and fever. In the second stage, which usually lasts two to three weeks, severe coughing attacks occur during the night, and then later during the day and night. The attacks can lead to inadequate oxygen, which can cause convulsions. During this stage death can occur. In the final stage, coughing lessens and recovery begins. Full recovery may take two to three months. The disease is rarely fatal.[304] However, when infants under six months contract pertussis, it can be serious and life-threatening. There is no specific treatment for pertussis. Antibiotics and cough suppressants have been used, but with little effect, and are generally not recommended. A vaccine against pertussis has been available since 1936 (and was put into general use during the 1940s).

Findings: The incidence and severity of whooping cough had begun to decline long before the pertussis vaccine was introduced.[305] From 1900 to 1935, the death rate from pertussis in the United States and England had already declined on its own by 79 percent and 82 percent, respectively (Figure 14).[306]

A study published in the *Journal of Pediatrics* indicates that the pertussis vaccine may be only 40-45 percent effective.[307] Further evidence indicates that immunity is not sustained. Susceptibility to pertussis 12 years after full vaccination may be as high as 95 percent.[308] For example, 2,187 cases of pertussis were reported to the CDC in 1984. Of the 560 patients aged seven months to six years with known vaccination status, nearly half (46 percent) had received vaccine protection.[309] In 1986, 1300 cases of pertussis were reported in Kansas. Of the patients with known vaccination status, 90 percent were "adequately" vaccinated.[310] And in 1993, during a pertussis outbreak in Ohio, 82 percent of younger children stricken with the disease had received regular doses of the vaccine (Figure 15).[311]

The diphtheria, tetanus, and pertussis vaccines are usually combined into a single formula (DTP or DTaP). Components of this triple shot (including the "newly formulated" and recently updated version) are "stabilized" using formaldehyde—a known carcinogen. Each dose also contains thimerosal—a derivative of mercury—and aluminum potassium sulfate.[312] Mercury and aluminum are toxic to humans.[313]

The United States never conducted its own clinical tests to determine whether the pertussis vaccine is safe and effective. Instead, it relies on data collected by Great Britain during the 1950s on children between six months and one-and-a-half years of age. Even though 42 of these children had convulsions within 28 days, 80 percent of the babies were 14 months of age or older, and the tests were designed to measure the efficacy (not safety) of the vaccine,

Figure 14:

The Pertussis Death Rate was Decreasing on its Own *Before* the Vaccine was Introduced

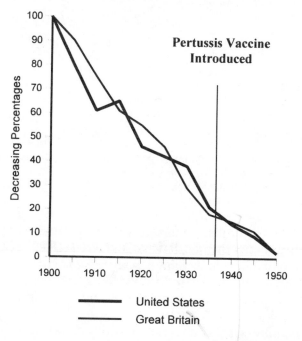

Copyright © 2002, Neil Z. Miller

From 1900 to 1935, *before* the pertussis vaccine was introduced, the death rate from pertussis in the United States and England had already declined on its own by 79 percent and 82 percent, respectively. Source: *International Mortality Statistics* (1981) by Michael Alderson.

U.S. health authorities use these results as evidence that the vaccine is safe to give to babies as young as six weeks of age. In fact, a two month old baby weighing less than ten pounds receives the same dose of pertussis vaccine as a 50 pound child entering preschool.[314]

The pertussis vaccine was used in animal experiments to help produce anaphylactic shock, and to cause an acute autoimmune encephalomyelitis (allergic encephalitis).[315] Post-vaccinal encephalitis may be the greatest cause of developmental and learning disabilities in the country today.[316] Scientists also developed an indirect test

Figure 15:
Pertussis Outbreak:
82% Were Vaccinated

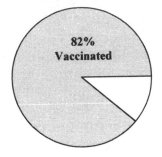

Copyright © 2002, Neil Z. Miller

During a pertussis outbreak in Ohio, 82 percent of younger children stricken with the disease had received regular doses of the vaccine. Source: *New England Journal of Medicine* (July 7, 1994):16-20.

---

to determine the efficacy and safety of the pertussis vaccine. If it rendered immunity in mice, it was considered effective in children. If the mice did not lose weight, it was presumed to be nontoxic.[317]

The pertussis vaccine may cause fever as high as 106 degrees, pain, swelling, diarrhea, projectile vomiting, excessive sleepiness, high-pitched screaming (not unlike the so-called cri encephalique, or encephalitic scream associated with central nervous system damage), inconsolable crying bouts, seizures, convulsions, collapse, shock, breathing problems, brain damage, and sudden infant death syndrome (SIDS).[318,319] In one report, serious reactions (including grand mal epilepsy and encephalopathy) were shown to be as high as one in 600.[320] In another study, it was reported that out of 15,752 shots administered to children, only 18 serious reactions (shock-collapse or convulsions) occurred (1 in 875). However, each child in the study received three to five shots. Thus, approximately one out of every 200 children who received the full DPT series suffered severe reactions.[321]

In 1994, the *Journal of the American Medical Association* published data showing that children diagnosed with asthma were five times more likely than not to have received the pertussis vaccine.[322] In 2000, a new study confirmed earlier findings that children who receive DPT or tetanus vaccines are significantly more likely to develop a "history of asthma" or other "allergy-related respiratory symptoms" than those who remain unvaccinated.[323]

Sudden Infant Death Syndrome (SIDS): Babies die at a rate seven times greater than normal within three days after getting a pertussis shot.[324,325] The three primary doses of pertussis are given to infants at two months, four months, and six months. Approximately 85 percent of SIDS cases occur in the period one through six months, with the peak incidence at age two to four months.[326]

In a recent scientific study of SIDS, episodes of apnea (cessation of breathing) and hypopnea (abnormally shallow breathing) were measured before and after pertussis vaccinations. *Cotwatch* (a sophisticated microprocessor placed under the baby's mattress to measure precise breathing patterns) was used, and the computer printouts it generated (in integrals of the "weighted apnea-hypopnea density") were analyzed. The data clearly shows that vaccination caused an extraordinary increase in episodes where breathing either nearly ceased or stopped completely (Figure 16). These episodes continued for months following vaccinations. Dr. Viera Scheibner, the author of the study, concluded that "vaccination is the single most prevalent and most preventable cause of infant deaths."[327-329]

In another study of 103 children who died of SIDS, Dr. William Torch found that more than two-thirds had been vaccinated with pertussis prior to death. Of these, 6.5 percent died within 12 hours of vaccination; 13 percent within 24 hours; 26 percent within three days; and 37, 61, and 70 percent within one, two, and three weeks, respectively (Figure 17). He also found that SIDS frequencies have a bimodal peak occurrence at two and four months—the same ages when initial doses of pertussis are administered to infants.[330]

The following excerpt is from a statement made by a distraught grandmother testifying before Congress regarding vaccine injury compensation:

"My name is Donna Gary. Our family should have celebrated our very first granddaughter's first birthday last month. Instead, we will commemorate the anniversary of her death at the end of this month.

"Our granddaughter, Lee Ann, was just eight weeks old when her mother took her to the doctor for her routine checkup. That included, of course, her first DPT inoculation and oral polio vaccine.

"In all her entire eight weeks of life this lovable, extremely alert baby had never produced such a blood-curdling scream as she did at the moment the shot was given. Neither had her mother ever

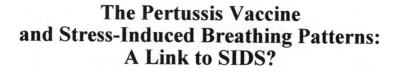

Figure 16:

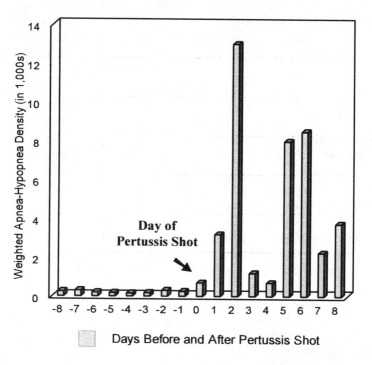

The Pertussis Vaccine and Stress-Induced Breathing Patterns: A Link to SIDS?

Weighted Apnea-Hypopnea Density (in 1,000s)

Day of Pertussis Shot

Days Before and After Pertussis Shot

Copyright © 2002, Neil Z. Miller

This chart represents a 17-day record of one child's breathing patterns before and after receiving the pertussis vaccine. Values above 1000 indicate acute stress-induced breathing. The author of this study concluded that "vaccination is the single most prevalent and most preventable cause of infant deaths." Source: *Vaccination: 100 Years of Orthodox Research...* by Dr. Viera Scheibner (Blackheath, Australia, 1993): 59-70, 225-235.

---

before seen her back arch as it did while she screamed. She was inconsolable. Even her daddy could not understand Lee Ann's uncharacteristic screaming and crying.

"Four hours later Lee Ann was dead. 'Crib death,' the doctor said—'SIDS.' 'Could it be connected to the shot?' her parents

Figure 17:

The Pertussis Vaccine and Sudden Infant Death Syndrome

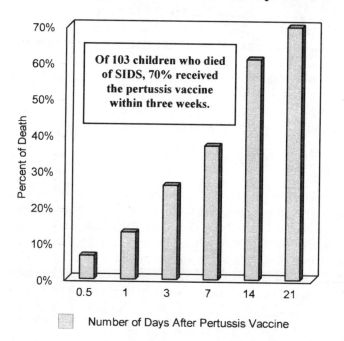

Of 103 children who died of SIDS, 70% received the pertussis vaccine within three weeks.

Number of Days After Pertussis Vaccine

Copyright © 2002, Neil Z. Miller

In a study of 103 children who died of SIDS, more than two-thirds had been vaccinated with pertussis prior to death. Of these, 6.5 percent died within 12 hours of vaccination; 13 percent within 24 hours; 26 percent within three days; and 37, 61, and 70 percent within one, two, and three weeks, respectively. Source: American Academy of Neurology, 34th Annual Meeting: *Neurology* 32(4).

---

implored. 'No.' 'But she just had her first DPT shot this afternoon. Could there possibly be any connection to it?' 'No, no connection at all,' the emergency room doctor said definitely.

"My husband and I hurried to the hospital the following morning after Lee Ann's death to talk with the pathologist before the autopsy. We wanted to make sure he was alerted to her DPT inoculation such a short time before her death—just in case there was something else he could look for to make the connection. He was unavailable to talk with us. We waited two-and-a-half hours. Finally, we got to talk to another doctor after the autopsy had been completed. He said it was 'SIDS.'

"In the months before Lee Ann was born I regularly checked with a friend as to the state of her grandchild's condition. He is nearly a year-and-a-half older than Lee Ann. On his first DPT shot he passed out cold for 15 minutes, right in the pediatrician's office. 'Normal reaction for some children,' the pediatrician reassured. The parents were scared, but they knew what a fine doctor they had. They trusted his judgment.

"When it was time for the second shot they asked, 'Are you sure it's all right? Is it really necessary?'

"Their pediatrician again reassured them. He told them how awful it was to experience, as he had, one of his infant patient's bout with whooping cough. That baby had died.

"They gave him his second DPT shot that day. He became brain-damaged.

"This past week I had an opportunity to read through printed copies of the hearings of this committee. I am dismayed to learn that this same talk has been going on for years, and nothing has progressed to incorporate what seems so obvious and necessary to keep from destroying any more babies, and to compensate financially those who have already been damaged for life.

"How accurate are our statistics on adverse reactions to vaccines when parents have been told, are still being told, 'No connection to the shot, no connection at all?'

"What about the mother I have recently talked with who has a four-year-old brain-damaged son? On all three of his DPT shots he had a convulsion in the presence of the pediatrician. 'No connection,' the pediatrician assured.

"I talked with a father in a town adjoining ours whose son died at the age of nine weeks, several months before our own granddaughter's death. It was the day after his DPT inoculation. 'SIDS' is the statement on the death certificate.

"Are the statistics that the medical world loves to quote to say, 'There is no connection,' really accurate, or are they based on poor diagnoses, poor recordkeeping?

"What is being done to provide a safer vaccine? Who is overseeing? Will it be the same scientists and doctors who have been overseeing in the past? How are physicians and clinics going to be held accountable to see that parents are informed of the possible reactions? And how are those children who should not receive the vaccine to be identified before they are damaged—or dead?

"Today is the National Day of Prayer. My prayer is that this committee be instrumental in doing what needs to be done—and soon. May there not be yet another year pass by with more children afflicted, and some dead, because those who can do so refuse to 'make the right connection.'"[331]

ACELLULAR PERTUSSIS (DTaP)

In 1981, Japan began giving their children a new "acellular" pertussis vaccine. They claimed it was less toxic and more effective than the standard "whole-cell" vaccine used in the United States. Many authorities in this country agreed, but claimed that the additional cost to produce the vaccine, and the logistics involved, did not justify making the switch.[332]

Findings: Japan reported a significant drop in serious reactions following use of the acellular vaccine. However, in 1975, a few years before the new pertussis vaccine was introduced in Japan, authorities raised the age of vaccination to two years. In the U.S., pertussis shots are begun at two months, and are continued throughout the infant's early, and high risk, months. Thus it has been difficult to ascertain whether the acellular vaccine is truly safer.[333]

In 1987, 66 victims of the Japanese pertussis vaccine won huge awards from their government. The court recognized that the authorities were denying reactions and the damaged plaintiffs were victimized so that the "public interest in preventing contagious diseases" wouldn't be undermined.[334]

In 1988, the United States tested the acellular pertussis vaccine on Swedish children. Efficacy with a two dose regimen was 69 percent. Several children died during the study. Ironically, U.S. health officials—who were indifferent to pursuing alternatives to their imperfect whole-cell vaccine—played coy by calling for more research into the deaths, even though they occurred up to five months after vaccination, causes included heroin intoxication, and Swedish officials concluded they were unrelated to the vaccinations. Deaths that occur within hours or days of a whole-cell vaccination in the U.S. are quickly dismissed and rarely investigated.[335,336]

In 1989, *Pediatrics* published a study showing that the acellular vaccine caused fewer of the mild-type reactions than the standard DPT vaccine. However, serious reactions, such as encephalitis, occurred at a higher rate than with the standard shot. Brain inflammation struck at the rate of one of every 106 vaccinated children.[337]

In 1992, the American Academy of Pediatrics (AAP) recommended replacing the standard whole-cell pertussis vaccine (DPT) with the acellular (DTaP) vaccine for the 4th and 5th doses only.[338] In 1996, U.S. authorities replaced DPT with the DTaP vaccine for all five doses—despite the contention by some researchers that "most of the mild and serious reactions which have been reported following DPT vaccination have also been reported following DTaP..."[339]

The following adverse reactions are typical of the unsolicited email received by the _Thinktwice Global Vaccine Institute_. (For more information, visit www.thinktwice.com)

"My son is one year old. On his nine-month visit, he received the DTaP shot. The next two days he was doing a strange sort of jerking movement with his face that I'd never seen before. It looked like a mini-seizure. His body would tighten up when they would occur. I am now worried about getting the next DTaP shot."

"My youngest daughter had a 'mild' reaction to the DPT. Her fever lasted three to four days, and she was cranky for a few weeks. My doctor suggested 1/2 dose for the next round; she had no reaction at all. Then we moved and her new pediatrician stated that 1/2 doses aren't recognized as a valid vaccination, but suggested the DTaP. Within hours she started to get a high fever, black diarrhea, and vomited. I called the doctor immediately, who stated this is a normal reaction. However, within a month her hair started falling out. I took her back to the doctor who told me to stop putting her hair into ponytails, that I was pulling her hair too tight. Well, it has been two years since, and her hair has finally grown back enough for very small ponytails. I am not going to get her vaccinated again."

"They gave my daughter the DTaP at three months after they told me there were no known side effects. I objected to her having the shot but they told me that they would call Child Protection Services if I refused to let her have the vaccine. Being a teenage parent, the fear of losing her loomed over me 24 hours a day, and I didn't want to make it a reality. So, I agreed to let her have it. Within minutes of arriving home she began to scream like I had never heard before. It scared me. She screamed for about 16 hours, with no break. The doctor swore that she was okay and was just "colicky." After 16 hours of screaming she became lethargic. She wouldn't even look up when I said her name, which she had always done before. She went into a seizure and ended up in the emergency room. My daughter now receives only the DT shot, and although the pediatrician's nurses get angry with me, I insist that I see the label of the shot bottle before any injections are given to her."[340]

HEPATITIS B

Hepatitis B is a viral infection. Symptoms may be similar to the flu, including weakness, loss of appetite, diarrhea, pain in the upper right abdomen, and jaundice (yellowing of the eyes and skin). In some cases, individuals who contract this disease may be carriers of the virus yet exhibit few or none of these symptoms. Acute hepatitis B usually runs its course within one year. Long-term or chronic infections may progress to liver failure, coma, and death.

In 1981, the Food and Drug Administration (FDA) licensed a plasma-derived hepatitis B vaccine. It contained hepatitis B antigens (disease matter) extracted from individuals infected with the disease. This vaccine was later withdrawn from the market because vaccines derived from human blood are capable of transmitting unforeseen and potentially dangerous viruses. (Several studies investigated the probability that recipients of the plasma-derived hepatitis B vaccine received vaccines contaminated with HIV, a precursor to AIDS.)[341,342] In 1986, the first of several genetically engineered (synthetic recombinant) vaccines was licensed for use on the general population.

Findings: The groups at highest risk of contracting hepatitis B are intravenous drug users, prostitutes, and sexually active gay men. Infants and children rarely develop this disease. In fact, less than one percent of all cases occur in children younger than 15 years.[343] In North America, Europe and Australia, true carriers of the virus represent just one-tenth of one percent of the population.[344]

Infants born to hepatitis B infected mothers have a greater chance of acquiring this disease. However, children are very unlikely to contract hepatitis B if the mother is not infected. Pregnant women may be screened for this disease if they are concerned.[345]

Studies claim that the hepatitis B vaccine provides immunity from the disease for five to ten years, but this conclusion contradicts the data. For example, in a study published in the *New England Journal of Medicine*, after five years antibody levels (presumed to correlate with immunity) declined sharply or no longer existed in 42 percent of the vaccine recipients. In addition, 34 of the 773 subjects (4.4 percent!) became infected with the virus.[346,347] In another study, fewer than 40 percent of the vaccine recipients had protective antibody levels after five years.[348] A similar study showed that 48 percent of the vaccine recipients had inadequate antibody levels after just four years.[349] In fact, according to the World Health Organization, up to "60 percent of adults will lose all detectable antibody to hepatitis B vaccine within 6 to 10 years."[350] The medical literature contains other case studies documenting vaccine failures.[351,352]

In 1991, the Centers for Disease Control and Prevention (CDC) recommended that all infants receive the hepatitis B vaccine. Today, a majority of states mandate this vaccine. Yet, surveys in medical journals indicate that up to 87 percent of pediatricians and family practitioners do not believe this vaccine is needed by their newborn patients (Figure 18).[353,354] Nevertheless, because high risk groups are difficult to reach, or have rejected this vaccine, and since children are "accessible," many now receive the complete series beginning at birth. Due to waning efficacy or partial immunity, older children are compelled to receive booster doses as well.

Authorities often claim that hospital employees are likely to contract and spread hepatitis B. They use this as a rationale for mandating the shot. However, in one study of 624 health workers, the risk of contracting hepatitis B was associated with the frequency of contact with blood, but did not correlate with the frequency of contact with patients. The authors concluded that health workers may become naturally immunized rather than infected through continuous exposure to low levels of hepatitis B.[355]

Adverse reactions following the plasma-derived and the synthetic recombinant hepatitis B vaccines have been noted in the scientific literature. These include diabetes, multiple sclerosis, Guillain-Barré syndrome, Bell's palsy, Rolf's Palsy, ocular and brachial plexus neuropathy, optic neuritis, central nervous system demyelination, lumbar reticulopathy, transverse myelitis, autoimmune reactions, thrombocytopenic purpura, anaphylaxis, arthritis, fever, headaches, pain, vomiting, vertigo, herpes zoster, and convulsions. Many of these reactions occurred after just one dose of the vaccine.[356-371]

This section contains unsolicited adverse reaction reports associated with the hepatitis B vaccine. They are typical of the daily emails received by the _Thinktwice Global Vaccine Institute._

"Our daughter was born healthy but we allowed her to get the hepatitis B vaccine, and at three days old she started having seizures. After a week in the local children's hospital surrounded by the best doctors and nurses, they said she had suffered a stroke."

"I am a mother of three boys—six years, four years, and almost seven months. But the problem with my family is, we no longer have our seven month old baby. We lost our dear baby when he was almost two months old. He passed away after receiving just one shot of the hepatitis B vaccine!"

"My son received the hepatitis B vaccine. Within days he had

Figure 18:

The Hepatitis B Vaccine:
Do Doctors Think it is Necessary?

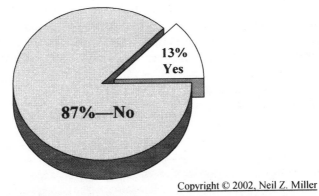

13%
Yes

87%—No

Copyright © 2002, Neil Z. Miller

Surveys in medical journals indicate that up to 87 percent of pediatricians and family practitioners do not believe the hepatitis B vaccine is needed by their newborn patients. Source: *Pediatrics* 1993; 91:699-702. *Journal of Family Practice* 1993; 36:153-57.

---

cold and flu-like symptoms. It quickly escalated into a high fever with itchy, red hives all over his body, with severe joint pain and swelling. He was hospitalized within 10 days of the shot. He is now diagnosed with juvenile rheumatoid arthritis and is on several medications. Prior to the shot he was a very healthy, active boy who played sports."

"After the nurse injected my 11-year-old daughter with her second hepatitis B shot, she got up, almost tripped into the next room, and fell flat to the ground. I went to pick her up not knowing what had happened, and when I lifted her up she was lifeless, and then her body started to shake. It was very frightening. She had passed out, and when she hit the floor her chin was bleeding and she had to get six stitches. The doctor said that she just passed out, but I am concerned about why she shook the way she did. I am scared to death to get her third shot."

"My 14 year old daughter had a toxic reaction to her hepatitis B vaccinations. Prior to the vaccines, my daughter competed in the National Junior Olympics and has always been an 'A' student. This has changed. She currently is suffering from chronic fatigue, dizziness, memory loss and sore joints. We have put her through a series of medical tests. She has evidence of autoimmune disease. The recommendation is to treat her with immuno-suppressive drugs or intravenous gammaglobulin. This is her life. I am very concerned. It breaks my heart. I write this with tears in my eyes. Please help."

"Ever since I received the hepatitis B vaccine I have had weakness and heaviness in my legs, among other symptoms. I've seen several doctors and had many tests to determine what is wrong with me. I fall in the category of multiple sclerosis-like symptoms."

"I was forced to receive the hepatitis B vaccine because my job placed me at 'high' risk. At first I experienced weird symptoms, then developed multiple sclerosis."[372]

CHICKENPOX

Chickenpox, or varicella, is a contagious disease caused by a virus. The technical name for this virus is varicella-zoster, a member of the herpes virus family. Chickenpox is considered by many experts to be a relatively harmless childhood disease.[373] Symptoms include a fever, runny nose, sore throat, and an itchy skin rash which can appear anywhere on the body. The rash and disease usually disappear after one or two weeks. The disease confers permanent immunity; the child will not contract it again.

A chickenpox vaccine has been available since the 1970s, but authorities were reluctant to license and promote it because the disease is rarely dangerous and confers lifelong immunity. Still, in 1995 the chickenpox vaccine was licensed for use in the U.S., and has been added to the list of "mandatory" shots in several states.

Findings: Chickenpox can be itchy and uncomfortable for a few days. Serious problems are rare. In fact, before a chickenpox vaccine was introduced, doctors used to recommend exposing your child to the virus, and parents organized "chickenpox parties," because complication rates increase when the disease is contracted by teenagers or adults.[374] Every year, of the millions of people who contract this disease, about 50 die from related complications.[375] Many of these are in adults who did not have chickenpox as a child, or in previously unhealthy children with already weakened immune systems from other diseases, such as AIDS, leukemia, or cancer.[376]

Prior to licensing the chickenpox vaccine, an important study concluded that a national chickenpox vaccination campaign would shift the age distribution of chickenpox cases from children, who are not likely to experience problems with this disease, to teenagers and adults, who have higher complication rates.[377] Yet, this did not stop authorities from licensing and mandating this vaccine, because "the U.S. could save five times as much as it would spend" on this shot by avoiding the costs incurred by moms and dads who stay home to care for their sick children.[378]

Efficacy rates for the chickenpox vaccine have not been reliably established. The vaccine is not effective in children under 12 months, and in all pre-licensure trials some vaccinated children contracted chickenpox.[379,380] "Vaccine failures" and/or the development of a rash virtually indistinguishable from chickenpox, account for many of the documented (and undocumented) complaints associated with this shot.[381-383] According to an FDA report, approximately 1 in 10 vaccinated children develop "breakthrough disease" following exposure to chickenpox.[384] Actual figures are worse because some people do not report their reactions, and because vaccinated children who contract shingles or some other disease as a result of the shot are not listed as recipients of an ineffective or failed vaccine.

When the chickenpox vaccine was first licensed, product inserts from a chickenpox vaccine manufacturer contained a warning that vaccinated individuals "may" be capable of transmitting the vaccine virus to close contacts, and that vaccine recipients "should avoid close association with susceptible high risk individuals" such as newborns, pregnant women, and immuno-compromised individuals.[385] A recent study published in the *Journal of Pediatrics* confirmed that vaccinated children can spread the disease.[386] Recently published federal data includes numerous cases of these "unintentional exposures." As a result, the CDC and FDA had to admit that "secondary transmission of the virus can occur."[387] Today, product labels for the chickenpox vaccine list "secondary transmission" of the vaccine virus as a known adverse event.[388,389] In other words, children vaccinated with the chickenpox shot are mobile carriers of the virus, and can spread this highly contagious disease to every susceptible person they come into contact with.

The FDA and CDC recently studied 6,574 reports of adverse reactions to the chickenpox vaccine and published their findings in the *Journal of the American Medical Association.*[390] Here is a summary of their findings: Adverse reactions in recipients of the chickenpox vaccine occurred at a rate of 67.5 reports per 100,000 doses sold. Approximately four percent of reports described "serious" adverse reactions. By FDA definition, "serious" reactions refer to

Figure 19:

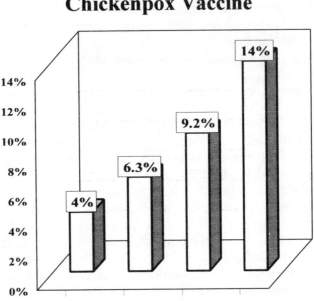

Serious Adverse Reactions: Chickenpox Vaccine

Serious adverse reaction rates (including numerous cases of neurological disorders, immune system damage, blood disorders, brain inflammation, seizures, and death) dramatically increase in younger age groups receiving the chickenpox vaccine. Source: *JAMA*, September 13, 2000.

Copyright © 2002, Neil Z. Miller

deaths, life-threatening events, hospitalizations, persistent or significant disabilities, and other incidents of medical importance. For example, the data analyzed in this review included numerous cases of neurological disorders, immune system damage, blood disorders, brain inflammation, seizures, and death.[391]

If we take the FDA analysis at face value, serious reactions to the chickenpox vaccine struck at a rate of four percent. This included victims in all age groups. However, children up to four years old had serious reactions at a rate of 6.3 percent; children up to two years old had serious reactions at a rate of 9.2 percent; and children vaccinated (by mistake) between birth and their first year of life had serious reactions at an astonishing rate of 14 percent! (Figure 19)[392]

The FDA and CDC findings included case histories. For example, a healthy 18-month-old boy who "had no history of allergy or any prior postvaccinal adverse event" before receiving the chickenpox vaccine (and others), was admitted to the intensive care unit four days later with a low platelet count. "He began to bleed from the mouth...and died two days later from cerebral hemorrhage."

Another child "without previous convulsions" had a seizure three days after varicella vaccine. Following his second dose one month later, he reacted with two tonic-clonic seizures. Researchers concluded, "This patient's positive rechallenge for seizure activity *increases suspicion that varicella vaccine may be more than a coincidental factor in observations of postvaccinal convulsions.* "[393]

The FDA and CDC findings also included numerous reports of vaccine recipients developing herpes zoster, or shingles, a painful skin eruption that can last for several weeks. This affliction can occur again and again, months or years following the shot. Once the varicella virus is injected into the body, it remains there indefinitely and can reactivate when immunity declines. According to Dr. Dennis Klinman of the FDA's Center for Biologics Evaluation and Research, and the author of a 2000 study published in *Nature Medicine*, reactivation of the latent infection can occur following vaccination with the live attenuated varicella zoster virus (chickenpox vaccine). "As immunity declines, the latent virus wakes up."[394,395] Earlier studies, including one published in the *New England Journal of Medicine*, already showed this link between the chickenpox vaccine and herpes zoster.[396,397]

Additional corroboration of vaccine-induced shingles can be found in the following personal stories typical of the unsolicited email received by the *Thinktwice Global Vaccine Institute:*

"I made the foolish decision to get my daughter the chickenpox vaccine. Within a few days she had an outbreak of pox. Now, a year later, she has another outbreak but I can't convince a doctor since she's supposedly immune due to the shot."

"My twins were immunized with the chickenpox vaccine. Ever since they received the shot, they have had a recurring rash that looks like chickenpox. It first showed up three days after vaccinations. Nothing works to treat the bumps. The bumps are concentrated in one area, typical of shingles. Our doctors deny it, so basically we just have to deal with this. I wish I had never vaccinated them against chickenpox. My other children caught chickenpox naturally and it never hurt any of them. Please pass this letter on to others who are considering this vaccine so they can make a better decision."[398]

HAEMOPHILUS INFLUENZAE TYPE B (HIB)

Haemophilus influenzae type b, or Hib (no relation to the flu), is a serious bacterial infection that can cause meningitis, pneumonia, swelling of the throat, and other disease complications. Hib is spread through sneezing, coughing, and secretions from an infected person. Treatment mainly consists of intravenously administered antibiotics. Oxygen therapy and other medical tactics may also be required.

In 1985, the first of several Hib vaccines was licensed for use in the U.S. This vaccine was ineffective in children under age two, so it was quickly recommended for all children two years old or older—even though 75 percent of all Hib cases occur *before* the age of two years.[399-403] From 1987 to 1990, several new "conjugated" Hib vaccines were licensed. By 1991, Hib vaccines were recommended for use in infants as young as two months.[404-406]

Findings: During the 1970s and 1980s, there were an estimated 16,000 to 20,000 Hib infections per year in the U.S.[407,408] Meningitis (inflammation of the membranes surrounding the brain and spinal cord) occurred in about half of the cases.[409] Around 25 percent of all Hib infections caused hearing loss, neurological problems, or pneumonia.[410-412] Inflammation of the throat accounted for nearly 15 percent of cases.[413] The mortality rate was about four percent.[414,415]

Hib infections occurred at a much lower rate during the 1940s and 1950s. In fact, Hib rates jumped 400 percent between 1946 and 1986[416-418]—a period coinciding with mass use of the DPT vaccine. Several factors appear to implicate this highly reactive combination shot.[419-423] Rates tumbled beginning in the 1990s, with just 329 cases of Hib in American children under five years of age in 1994, 259 cases in 1995, and 144 cases in 1996 and 1997 combined.[424-426]

Sixty percent of all Hib cases occur in children less than 12 months of age; 90 percent occur in children less than five years old.[427] Native American Indians, Eskimo children, African-Americans, and children from lower socioeconomic families are all at increased risk of contracting Hib.[428-429] In the U.S., African-American children are four times as likely to contract Hib as white children.[430]

Children are at risk of contracting Hib disease following their Hib vaccinations. Doctors have been warned by the CDC that cases may occur after vaccination, "prior to the onset of the protective effects of the vaccine."[431] Studies warn of "increased susceptibility" to the disease during the first seven days after vaccination.[432] The

American Academy of Pediatrics has warned doctors to look for signs of the disease in children following vaccination.[433] In fact, several studies found that Hib-vaccinated children are up to six times more likely than non-Hib-vaccinated children to contract Hib during the first week following vaccination.[434-438] In one study of children who contracted Hib at least three weeks after their shot, more than 70 percent developed meningitis.[439] Additional research has confirmed that antibody levels *decline* rather than increase immediately following Hib vaccinations[440,441] —even with the newer conjugated Hib vaccines[442] —placing the child at greater risk for invasive disease.

Here is a letter from a distraught mother confirming an increased susceptibility to the disease following vaccination:

"My daughter was born a healthy baby girl and was progressing great. Then I got a vaccine reminder in the mail. I made an appointment, got her shots, and one week later my daughter was dead. The autopsy report stated: 'Haemophilus influenzae.' She was not ill in any way, but now my baby is dead. They keep saying it can't happen, but what more proof do they need? I have a dead baby who died of the disease that she was supposed to be immune to."[443]

Hib vaccines are often given simultaneously with other vaccines. Some drug companies combine the Hib vaccine with DTaP. Thus, when a child has an adverse reaction to the shot, it is often difficult to ascertain which component of the vaccine (or of the several simultaneously administered vaccines) was responsible. Nevertheless, the medical literature contains numerous reports confirming likely correlations between the Hib vaccine and serious ailments, including: Guillain-Barré syndrome, transverse myelitis (paralysis of the spinal cord), aseptic meningitis, invasive pneumococcal disease, thrombocytopenia (a decrease in blood platelets leading to internal bleeding), erythema multiforme, fever, rash, hives, vomiting, diarrhea, seizures, convulsions, and sudden infant death syndrome.[444-451]

The Hib vaccine may also be linked to new epidemics of diabetes. Sharp increases of insulin-dependent diabetes mellitus have been recorded in the USA, England, and other European countries following mass immunization campaigns with the Hib vaccine.[452,453] In a landmark study published in the *British Medical Journal,* more than 200,000 Finnish children were split into three groups.[454,455] The first group received no doses of the Hib vaccine. The second group received one dose of the Hib vaccine (at 24 months of age). The third group received four doses of the Hib vaccine (at 3, 4, 6, and 18 months of age). At ages seven and ten, the total number of cases of type 1 diabetes in all three groups was tallied.

Figure 20:

The Hib Vaccine and Rising Diabetes Rates

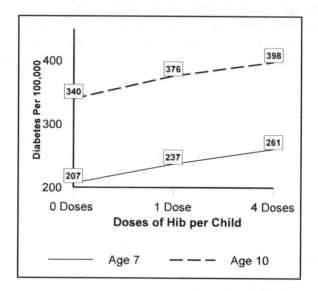

Copyright © 2002, Neil Z. Miller

More than 200,000 Hib-vaccinated and non-vaccinated children were compared. One group received no doses; another group received 1 dose; the third group received four doses of the Hib vaccine. At ages seven and ten, the number of cases of type 1 diabetes in all three groups was tallied. At age seven, there were 54 more cases per 100,000 children in the group that received four doses of the Hib vaccine vs. the group that received no doses—a 26% increase. At age ten, there were 58 more cases per 100,000 children in the group that received four doses vs. the group that received no doses. According to some experts, "the potential risk of the vaccine exceeds the potential benefit." Source: *British Medical Journal,* October 23, 1999.

Results: At age seven, there were 54 more cases per 100,000 children in the group that received four doses of the Hib vaccine when compared to the group that received no doses—a 26 percent increase![456,457] At age ten, there were 58 more cases per 100,000 children in the group that received four doses of the Hib vaccine when compared to the group that received no doses (Figure 20).[458] Based on an annual birth rate of about 4 million children, in the U.S. alone this translates into 2,300 additional (and avoidable) cases of diabetes every year.[459] (Each case of insulin dependent diabetes is estimated to cost more than $1 million in medical costs and lost productivity.)[460] By contrast, the Hib vaccine is expected to prevent a much smaller number of severe disabilities.[461] These figures depict significant differences, and according to some experts who analyzed the data, a causal relationship between the Hib vaccine and type 1 diabetes is supported.[462] Furthermore, "the increased risk of diabetes in the vaccinated group exceeds the expected decreased risk of complications of Hib meningitis."[463] Thus, these experts issued a warning to the public that, in their estimation, "the potential risk of the vaccine exceeds the potential benefit."[464]

Personal stories by concerned parents confirm that the vaccine may be more detrimental than beneficial:

"I have a son who was diagnosed with diabetes six months after his first Hib shot. Two of his friends were also diagnosed six months after their first Hib shot. There is no history of diabetes in any of these families."

"Our 10-year-old daughter was diagnosed with diabetes [a few months after she received her Hib vaccine]."

"My daughter received a Hib vaccine a few months before she was diagnosed with type 1 diabetes."[465]

PNEUMOCOCCAL DISEASE

Streptococcus pneumoniae, or pneumococcal disease, is a serious bacterial illness that can cause meningitis, pneumonia, ear infections, sinusitis, and bacteremia (an infection of the blood). The pneumococcal pathogen consists of approximately 90 different strains, including serogroups 1, 2, 3, 4, 5, 6B, 7F, 8, 9N, 9V, 10A, 11A, 12F, 18C, 19A, 26, 51, 54, 68, and so on.[466,467]

A vaccine containing 23 strains of the pneumococcal germ has been available for many years. Authorities recommend it for seniors and "high risk" children over age two[468,469] —even though studies show it to be ineffective at preventing pneumococcal infections.[470-472]

In 2000, the FDA approved a new vaccine— Prevnar® or PCV7—for children 23 months and younger.[473] It contains seven of the estimated 90 different pneumococcal strains and is given as a four dose series starting at two months of age (Figure 21).[474,475]

Findings: Most healthy children are not at risk from this disease. In fact, according to the Red Book Report of the Committee on Infectious Diseases published by the American Academy of Pediatrics, "[Pneumococcal infections in children] are more likely

Figure 21:

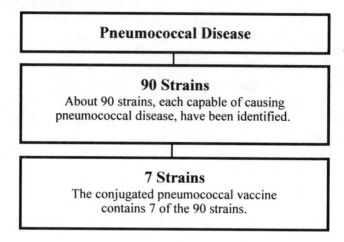

The conjugated pneumococcal vaccine contains seven of the approximately 90 pneumococcal strains capable of causing pneumococcal disease. Source: The vaccine manufacturer's package inserts.

Copyright © 2002, Neil Z. Miller

to occur when predisposing conditions exist, including immuno-globulin deficiency, Hodgkin's disease, congenital or acquired immunodeficiency (including HIV), nephrotic syndrome, some viral upper respiratory tract infections, splenic dysfunction, splenectomy and organ transplantation."[476]

Efficacy of the pneumococcal 7-valent conjugate vaccine (Prevnar®) was assessed based upon a study in which babies injected with the new vaccine were compared to babies injected with other vaccines.[477,478] A true controlled study comparing babies vaccinated with pneumococcus to non-vaccinated babies was never conducted.

In practical terms, it will be nearly impossible to tell how well the pneumococcal shot really works because its efficacy is only determined by its protection against bacterial disease caused by the seven strains included in the vaccine. This vaccine will not protect against pneumococcal disease caused by any of the several dozen other strains of streptococcus pneumoniae. Nor will this vaccine protect against bacterial infections caused by hemophilus influenzae type b or meningococcus.[479]

This conjugated pneumococcal vaccine is relatively new. No one will know for sure just how safe (or unsafe) it is until after it has been "tested" on millions of children. According to the American Academy of Pediatrics (AAP), "Available data suggest that PCV7 (Prevnar®) may prove to be among the most reactogenic vaccine of those currently used..."[480]

The package inserts produced by the vaccine manufacturer list several adverse reactions that occurred following trials of the vaccine. Although the manufacturer does not admit a causative relationship between this vaccine and many of these reactions, parents who are considering this vaccine may wish to weigh the implications. Such reactions included: asthma, seizures, pneumonia, diabetes, autoimmune disease, ear infections, neutropenia, thrombocytopenia, wheezing, croup, and sudden infant death syndrome.[481]

Personal stories confirm a probable link to adverse reactions: "My 6-month-old received Prevnar two days ago. She vomited that evening. The injection site is very inflamed. It looks like a burn [and] has a big knot under it that...extends from the site like a finger."

"My 10-month-old son received Prevnar four days ago. Since then he has been vomiting and developed a rash on his body. I will not let him receive the vaccine again."

"My 12-month-old daughter just received Prevnar [and other vaccines]. She vomited for three hours and had diarrhea. My baby was admitted to the hospital and diagnosed with pneumonia."[482]

MENINGOCOCCAL DISEASE

Neisseria meningitidis, or meningococcal disease, is a serious bacterial illness that can cause meningitis and meningococcemia, or septicaemia (blood poisoning). The meningococcal pathogen consists of at least 13 different strains, including serogroups A, B, C, Y, W-135, 29E, and Z.[483] Serogroup C (alternately referred to as Meningoccus C, MenC, or **Meningitis C**), accounts for about 20 percent of all cases of meningococcal disease in the United States and 40 percent of all cases in the United Kingdom (Figure 22).[484,485]

At least three new meningococcal vaccines were recently developed and recommended for babies as young as two months.

Findings: Infants under one year of age are at greatest risk of contracting meningococcus. Children aged 1-5 years are the next highest risk group. Teens 15-19 are more susceptible to this disease as well.[486] In 1998, Australia reported 421 cases of the disease, Canada had just 126 cases, and Japan made only six notifications.[487] In the United States, outbreaks of group C meningococcal disease

Figure 22:

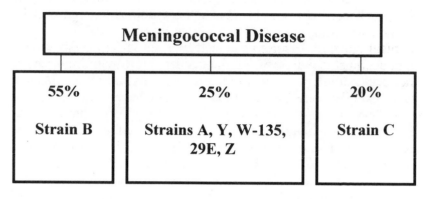

Copyright © 2002, Neil Z. Miller

80% of all meningococcal disease in the USA is caused by serogroups other than Strain C. Source: _Physician's Desk Reference,_ 53rd edition.

---

have been reported."[488] The CDC estimates that "between 100 and 125 cases of meningitis occur among U.S. college students annually and cause 5 to15 deaths."[489] However, no mention is made of the specific pathogen (a virus, Hib, pneumococcus, or meningococcus) responsible for these "estimated" cases of meningitis, nor does the CDC provide documentation to confirm their methods for making such estimates. The British Department of Health concedes that "Meningococcal infection is relatively rare, affecting approximately 5 in 100,000 people a year in the United Kingdom."[490]

No one can know for sure just how safe the meningococcal vaccine is until after it has been on the market for several years. A fact sheet produced by the British Department of Health flatly states that "No adverse effects of the vaccine have been seen."[491] Yet, by September 5, 2000, less than one year after a nationwide Meningitis C vaccination campaign was initiated, the British Committee on Safety of Medicines (CSM) had received 7,742 Yellow Card reports—suspected adverse reactions—following administration of this vaccine, including at least 12 deaths.[492] The British government tried to convince the public that most of the deaths were caused by sudden infant death syndrome.[493]

The Meningitis C vaccine is designed to protect against bacterial disease caused by the C strain of the meningococcus pathogen— just 20 percent of all cases in the U.S. and 40 percent in the U.K.[494]

The vaccine does not contain the B strain of meningococcus—the most frequent cause of the disease (Figure 22).[495] Nor is it possible for this vaccine to protect against bacterial disease caused by pneumococcus, haemophilus influenzae type b, or newly emerging atypical strains.[496] Thus, when a person is vaccinated and still contracts bacterial disease, it will be difficult to determine whether the vaccine failed or whether the disease was caused by the vaccine, by another strain, or by a completely different bacterial pathogen.

The following experience typifies the possibilities: "When I was in high school my parents had me vaccinated for meningitis. Following my vaccination, I ended up in the hospital with a major infection that attacked every area of my system. My parents told me that for the first two days that I was hospitalized I did not even recognize them. The doctors performed a lumbar puncture on me. This procedure involved freezing my mid-section so they could insert a large needle into the pit of my spinal cord to withdraw fluid for testing. Their diagnosis was meningitis. I remained hospitalized for three weeks. They did not want to even consider that my meningitis vaccination could have caused my nearly fatal disease."[497]

The position of the American Academy of Pediatrics is that "universal vaccination [with meningococcal vaccine] is not necessary."[498,499] The federal Advisory Committee on Immunization Practices conducted a financial analysis of vaccination for all college students and determined that it is not likely to be cost-effective for society as a whole because "the overall risk for meningococcal disease among college students is low" and college freshmen are only "at modestly increased risk for meningococcal disease relative to other persons their age."[500]

HEPATITIS A

Hepatitis A is a contagious liver disease usually transmitted through contaminated food or water. Symptoms may be similar to the flu, with fever, chills, and fatigue. Jaundice is common. In 1995, a hepatitis A vaccine was licensed in the United States.

Findings: According to the CDC, "the overall incidence of hepatitis A has declined in the United States over the past several decades primarily as a result of better hygienic and sanitary conditions."[501] In the early 1990s, about 12,000 cases were reported each year in the U.S.[502] Signs and symptoms usually last less than two months.[503] Complete recovery is typical.[504] However, the CDC estimates that in the U.S. about 100 people die each year from the disease.[505] Even so, the case-fatality rate among persons of all ages with acute hepatitis A is just .3 percent (less than one-third of one percent).[506] More than 70 percent of all hepatitis A deaths occur in adults greater than 50 years of age.[507]

The groups at highest risk of contracting hepatitis A are persons traveling to regions of the world where this disease is endemic, men who have sex with other men, and IV drug users. Children are _not_ among the groups at greatest risk.[508] Nevertheless, authorities believe that "routine vaccination of children is the most effective way to reduce hepatitis A incidence nationwide."[509] In other words, children will be subjected to all of the potential risks of a questionable vaccine, with little self-benefit, as part of an overall immunization strategy to protect high-risk groups whose members are difficult to reach or who may choose to reject the vaccine.

The hepatitis A vaccine is propagated in "human fibroblasts" originated from aborted fetal tissue. It contains formaldehyde (a known carcinogen), aluminum hydroxide, and 2-phenoxyethanol, a toxic chemical comparable to antifreeze.[510]

The hepatitis A vaccine is not covered by the National Vaccine Injury Compensation Program. Yet, many serious adverse events linked to this vaccine have been reported to the manufacturer. These include: anaphylaxis, Guillaine-Barré syndrome, brachial plexus neuropathy, transverse myelitis, encephalopathy, meningitis, erythema multiforme, and multiple sclerosis.[511] In addition, the Vaccine Adverse Event Reporting System (VAERS), operated by the CDC and FDA, receives numerous reports of "neurologic, hematologic, and autoimmune syndromes" linked to this vaccine.[512]

The duration of protection "is unknown at present."[513] Also, the incubation period (the time between being exposed and showing symptoms) of hepatitis A can be 50 days. Therefore, when a child receives the vaccine and contracts the disease shortly thereafter, the vaccine will not be implicated as defective or causative. Instead, the child will be blamed for harboring a pre-existing condition.[514]

RESPIRATORY SYNCYTIAL VIRUS (RSV)

Respiratory syncytial virus (RSV) is the most common cause of bronchiolitis and pneumonia among infants and children under one year of age.[515] It also causes severe respiratory illness in the elderly.[516] RSV is very contagious. Symptoms are initially similar to the common cold, then worsen as the infected person develops fever, wheezing, and difficulty breathing. Most healthy children recover in one to two weeks.[517,518] However, during their first RSV infection, about one percent of infants will require hospitalization.[519] Some people die from complications of the disease.[520]

Treatment of severe RSV infection is mainly supportive: oxygen therapy, hydration, and nutrition.[521] A vaccine does not yet exist. Researchers have been hampered by the mutable nature of the organism, and "early attempts [at developing a vaccine] actually made the disease worse on subsequent infection."[522] However, two "preventive agents" were licensed by the FDA. In 1996, Respigam, an immune globulin treatment made from human plasma, became available.[523] In 1998, Synagis,® a "monoclonal antibody" produced in human and mouse genes, entered the market.[524,525]

Findings: In 1956, respiratory syncytial virus (RSV) was discovered in chimpanzees.[526] According to Dr. Viera Scheibner, who studied more than 30,000 pages of medical papers dealing with vaccination, RSV viruses "formed prominent contaminants in polio vaccines, and were soon detected in children."[527] They caused serious cold-like symptoms in small infants and babies who received the polio vaccine.[528] In 1961, the *Journal of the American Medical Association* published two studies confirming a causal relationship between RSV and "relatively severe lower respiratory tract illness."[529,530] The virus was found in 57 percent of infants with bronchiolitis or pneumonia, and in 12 percent of babies with a milder febrile respiratory disease. Infected babies remained ill for three to five months.[531] RSV was also found to be contagious, and soon spread to adults where it has been linked to the common cold.[532] Today, children who are most at risk of serious complications from RSV include infants born prematurely or with chronic lung disease, immune system problems, neuromuscular disorders, congenital heart disease, and other pre-existing conditions.[533]

Synagis® is given as a series of five monthly injections at the start of and during the RSV season (usually November to April). It is very expensive; each injection may cost $900 or more.[534] One mother reported being charged more than $7,000 for a single dose and $2600 for each subsequent dose. Her insurance did not pay.[535]

Synagis® is indicated for the prevention of serious *lower* respiratory tract infections caused by RSV. Studies show that it will not alter the incidence and mean duration of hospitalization for non-RSV respiratory illness nor will it prevent *upper* respiratory tract infections.[536,537] In fact, clinical studies indicate that children receiving Synagis® are _more likely_ to experience upper respiratory tract infections than children who do not receive it.[538] Furthermore, some children will develop RSV despite having received Synagis.® The data suggests that their illnesses will be no less severe than children who develop RSV without Synagis.®[539]

In a controlled clinical study, Synagis® was found to increase the likelihood of developing otitis media (an ear infection), rhinitis, pharyngitis, rash, pain, and hernia.[540] Other adverse events reported in children receiving this "preventive" biotech commodity include: fever, cough, wheeze, bronchiolitis, pneumonia, bronchitis, asthma, croup, dyspnea, sinusitis, apnea, diarrhea, vomiting, liver function abnormality, viral infection, fungal dermatitis, eczema, seborrhea, conjunctivitis, anemia, flu syndrome, and failure to thrive.[541]

To learn more about vaccine safety, efficacy, laws,
support groups, natural alternatives,
reversing vaccine damage, and more,
please visit the...
Thinktwice Global Vaccine Institute
www.thinktwice.com

More Vaccines

The childhood vaccines previously covered represent just a few of the many that already exist or are in the developmental stages. For example, medical scientists are working on vaccines against cancer, AIDS, venereal disease, venoms, environmental toxins, and even the common cold. Scientists are also experimenting with a vaccine against pregnancy, vaccines crossbred into our food supply, and a time-released "supervaccine" containing disease matter from numerous remote ailments.[542,543]

If the principles behind the theory of vaccinations are flawed, future vaccines are probably doomed to failure as well. For example, according to Dr. Richard Moskowitz, the people that need an AIDS vaccine the most are already "seriously immunocompromised." Giving a suppressive vaccine to everyone would increase the odds of developing AIDS for those already at high risk. It would weaken the general population as well.[544,545]

This chapter contains information on the anthrax, smallpox, and flu vaccines. It also includes a section on multiple vaccines administered simultaneously.

ANTHRAX

Anthrax is a severe bacterial disease that primarily affects warm blooded animals, especially livestock. Humans can be infected as well. The disease is caused by the bacterium *Bacillus anthracis,* which produces spores that can remain dormant for years in soil and on animal products, such as hides, wool, hair, or bones.[546]

Animals get the disease by eating infected grass or carcasses, drinking infected water, or inhaling infected dust. They die suddenly with little or no symptoms.[547] *People* contract anthrax in one of three ways: 1) by coming into contact with the bacterium, or infected animals or animal products, 2) by inhaling airborne particles, or 3) by eating undercooked meat from diseased livestock (Figure 23).[548]

Figure 23:

How is Anthrax Contracted?

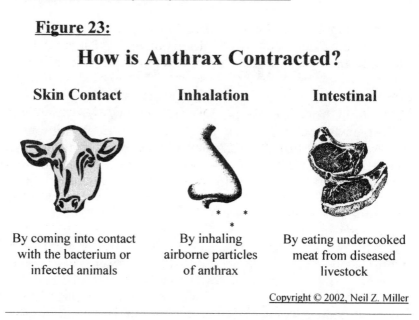

Skin Contact	Inhalation	Intestinal
By coming into contact with the bacterium or infected animals	By inhaling airborne particles of anthrax	By eating undercooked meat from diseased livestock

Copyright © 2002, Neil Z. Miller

In 1940, the Soviet Union developed the first anthrax vaccine for human use.[549] The United States and Great Britain produced human anthrax vaccines during the 1950s.[550] The currently available U.S. vaccine was formulated in the 1960s and licensed by the FDA in 1970, two years before efficacy data (scientific proof that it works) were required.[551,552] New anthrax vaccines are being developed.

Findings: Anthrax is rare; when it does occur, it is almost always an occupational hazard, contracted by those who sort wool or handle animal hides—farmers, butchers, and veterinarians. The disease is most often found in agricultural regions of South and Central America, eastern Europe, Asia, Africa, and the Middle East.[553] From 1900 to 1976, only 18 cases of the inhaled version were reported in the United States.[554] However, in 2001 anthrax was mailed to several media outlets and federal offices in the U.S. exposing numerous people to the disease.[555]

Symptoms usually appear within one week of exposure but vary depending upon how the disease is contracted:

1. Cutaneous anthrax is the most common, and mildest, form of the disease. This occurs through skin contact—when the bacteria enter a cut or wound. At first, an itchy raised area like an insect bite appears. Within one to two days, inflammation occurs and a blister forms around a black center of dying tissue. Other symptoms include shivering and chills. If bacteria spread to the nearest lymph gland, the disease can cause a form of blood poisoning that is fatal.

2. Inhalation or pulmonary anthrax occurs by inhaling the bacteria or bacterial spores. The disease begins with cold or flu-like symptoms—fever, fatigue, and headache—then progresses to bronchitis, pneumonia, and a state of shock. This rare form of anthrax is usually fatal.

3. Intestinal anthrax is caused by eating meat from an infected animal. The first signs are nausea and vomiting, loss of appetite, fever, and abdominal pain. It progresses to inflammation and ulcers of the stomach and intestines, vomiting of blood, and bloody diarrhea. This form of anthrax is also rare and often fatal.[556]

If caught early, anthrax is curable by administering high doses of penicillin.[557] Several antibiotics are effective against anthrax when it occurs naturally. Ciprofloxacin (Cipro) and doxycycline (Doxy) have been licensed by the FDA for use against all forms of the disease.[558] (Severe side effects are possible.)[559-563] Although cutaneous anthrax may be cured following a single dose of antibiotic, prolonged treatment is recommended. Victims of inhalation anthrax must take high doses of antibiotics for 60 days, starting immediately after exposure.[564] Some doctors use other regimens as well.

Anthrax is not considered contagious. There are no reports of the disease spreading from human to human. Thus, communicability is not likely when managing or visiting ill patients.[565] However, the prognosis for untreated anthrax is poor. About 20 percent of all unattended cutaneous cases will end in death. Most treated patients will recover.[566] All patients with inhalation anthrax will die if left untreated.[567] Only 10 percent will survive if treatment is postponed until symptoms appear and the spores have begun to release toxins.[568] Intestinal anthrax is fatal in about half the cases.[569]

In 1962, the *American Journal of Public Health* published the only randomized clinical study (Brachman, et al.) of a "protective-antigen anthrax vaccine."[570] Employees at four factories where anthrax-tainted goat hair was handled, were vaccinated. However, participants were only monitored for ill effects that occurred within two days of each shot, and adverse reaction rates within this limited time frame were not recorded. Nevertheless, the vaccine was touted as 92.5 percent effective.[571] According to Dr. Meryl Nass, a recognized expert on anthrax and biological warfare, "the actual percent efficacy cannot be calculated due to the small number of cases...five inhalation cases do not permit any conclusion about vaccine efficacy with regard to inhaled organisms."[572] Also, according to a March 2000 investigative report issued by the Institute of Medicine (IOM), vaccine research was terminated at one of the four factories (the largest of the study sites) after the initial series of three injections.[573] Data from this site is omitted from the study results, despite "a large number of systemic reactions."[574,575] The IOM report also noted that 81 subjects withdrew from the vaccine trials (at the other three factories) before completing the series of shots, yet data from these individuals was omitted from the study results as well.[576]

From 1986 to 1995, several studies tested the efficacy of the U.S. human anthrax vaccine on guinea pigs and mice. After the animals were vaccinated (typically with three shots, 2 to 3 weeks apart), they were exposed to several different strains of anthrax. Survival rates for vaccinated guinea pigs ranged from zero percent to 100 percent.[577-584] Survival rates for vaccinated mice ranged from zero percent to 10 percent.[585-587]

In 1993, the *Journal of Infectious Diseases* published a study in which monkeys were administered an anthrax vaccine shortly after being exposed to the disease. Survival rates were no better than in unvaccinated controls.[588] However, in 1996 U.S. army researchers published the results of a new study in which 25 adult rhesus monkeys received two injections of the human anthrax vaccine (two weeks apart). The monkeys were then exposed to the aerosolized spores of the Ames strain of anthrax at 8 weeks, 38 weeks, or 100 weeks. All of the vaccinated monkeys survived challenge at either 8 weeks or 38 weeks, and seven of eight monkeys survived challenge at 100 weeks.[589] Although the data in this study suggests that the U.S. human anthrax vaccine may protect adult rhesus monkeys against inhalation anthrax for up to two years, it is important to note that they were only exposed to a single strain of the disease. Researchers are currently aware of more than 1300 strains of anthrax.[590] The authors of this study also note that "immune mechanisms against inhalation anthrax may vary in different animal species." Thus, "these findings suggest...that the ability of the licensed human anthrax vaccine to stimulate cell-mediated immunity may be greater in some species than others."[591] Animals also differ from humans in their immunological responses. No one knows how animal studies of vaccine efficacy can be extrapolated to people. In fact, the scientists who conducted the study admit: "There is currently no known surrogate marker or in vitro correlate of immunity that allows direct comparison of immunity in humans to that in monkeys."[592]

In 1998, U.S. army researchers published another study in which rhesus monkeys were exposed to inhalation anthrax six weeks after being vaccinated with either the U.S. human anthrax vaccine or with experimental anthrax vaccines. The data showed that each vaccine provided "significant protection."[593] Authors of this study also noted that "results of recent studies show that anthrax vaccines vary in their efficacy among different species."[594] And like the earlier primate study, the monkeys were only exposed to a single strain of anthrax. Researchers did not test their vaccines against any of the other hundreds of strains circulating across the globe. However, in a recent *unpublished* study conducted by the Department of Defense (DoD), more than 20 different strains from around the world were tested against the U.S. human anthrax vaccine. Guinea pigs were vaccinated prior to being exposed to different strains of anthrax. Fourteen of the strains killed at least 75 percent of the vaccinated guinea pigs. Nine of the strains killed at least 85 percent of the rodents. Survival rates were even worse for strains found in Zimbabwe, Namibia, and France (Figure 24).[595]

Anthrax Vaccines Within the U.S. Military: Thousands of U.S. military personnel who served in the Persian Gulf War were forced to take an anthrax vaccine. Eighty-two percent received no written or verbal information about it; 76 percent could not refuse it; and 42 percent reported side effects after receiving it (Figure 25).[596] Many are incapacitated from debilitating ailments that range from bleeding rashes, gums, and sinuses, to muscle aches, swollen joints, chronic fatigue, diarrhea, hair loss, severe headaches, and memory loss. Over time, their symptoms became more acute. Many vets are now confined to wheelchairs and hospital beds.[597,598]

Despite the many lessons to be learned from the compulsory vaccine program inflicted on Gulf War veterans, on December 15, 1997, the U.S. military initiated a new plan to vaccinate all active duty personnel against anthrax. This "medical force protection effort" is called the Anthrax Vaccine Immunization Program (AVIP).[599] Shortly after it was instituted, veterans began complaining about debilitating illnesses following their shots. They were unable to decline the vaccine, and authorities refused to document adverse reactions. Eventually, the soldiers' complaints reached Congress, and from March 1999 through October 2000 several hearings were held to investigate the safety and efficacy of the DoD's AVIP.[600]

In one study submitted as evidence, "Evaluation of safety records show that one or more systemic symptoms occurred in 44 percent of recipients of vaccines within the first seven days after the booster

Figure 24:

U.S. Anthrax Vaccine:
Efficacy in Guinea Pigs
(Following Exposure to
Geographically Diverse Anthrax Strains)

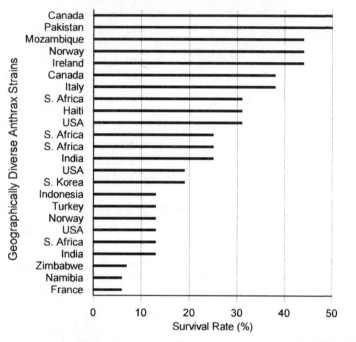

Copyright © 2002, Neil Z. Miller

Guinea pigs were vaccinated prior to being exposed to one of more than 20 different anthrax strains from around the world. Fourteen of the strains killed at least 75 percent of the vaccinated guinea pigs. Nine of the strains killed at least 85 percent of the rodents. Survival rates were even worse for strains found in Zimbabwe, Namibia, and France. Source: DoD; presented at the International Anthrax Conference (September 1998).

doses."[601] According to Dr. Meryl Nass, who testified before Congress regarding the dubious safety and efficacy of the mandatory anthrax vaccine, "Most important to the discussion we're having today is the question of whether service members currently being vaccinated are developing chronic, adverse effects from the anthrax vaccination... As a publicly known expert on anthrax vaccinations... I am sorry to report that the illness symptoms described to me are

Figure 25:

Gulf War Veterans and the Mandatory Anthrax Vaccine

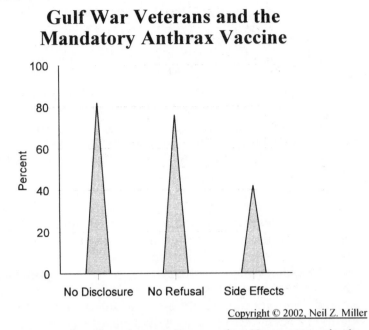

Copyright © 2002, Neil Z. Miller

Gulf War vets were forced to take an anthrax vaccine. 82 percent received no written or verbal information about it; 76 percent could not refuse it; 42 percent reported side effects after receiving it. Source: U.S. Senate (May 6, 1994).

---

remarkably similar, and also mimic the symptoms reported by numerous ill Gulf War veterans. This illness resembles Chronic Fatigue syndrome, with fatigue, sleep disturbance and cognitive deficits. There is a significant component of headache, muscle pain and joint pain, along with respiratory and abdominal complaints. In addition, many service members report neurologic symptoms including sensory neuropathies and widespread autonomic dysfunction. Many report sensory hypersensitivity, and some chemical sensitivity... Persisting symptoms have included...memory loss, cognitive disturbances, sleep disorders, peripheral sensory neuropathies, intermittent abdominal pain, diarrhea, chest pains, recurring rashes, blackouts or seizures."[602]

In summary, Dr. Nass also testified that "vaccines are unlikely to provide a robust defense against known biological agents and are even less likely to provide a defense against novel, genetically engineered agents... There is no good evidence for [anthrax] vaccine safety, efficacy or necessity."[603]

SMALLPOX

Smallpox is a highly contagious disease caused by the _variola_ virus. It is usually spread by inhaling droplets discharged from the nose and mouth of an infected person.[604] Smallpox can also be transmitted through infected blankets, linens and clothing.[605]

Symptoms begin 12 days after exposure to the virus: fever, nausea, vomiting, headache, back ache, and muscle pains. A rash develops on the whole body. As recovery begins, fever and other symptoms subside. The pustules crust over and may leave scars. The disease usually confers permanent immunity; the infected person will not contract it again.[606]

Antiviral medications and other drugs do not work to shorten the duration or alleviate the symptoms of smallpox. Treatment is focused on providing nutrition, increasing comfort, and reducing secondary infections. In addition, the patient is usually isolated from the public to prevent spread of the virus.[607]

A smallpox vaccine—often promoted as "pure lymph from the calf"—has been available since the early 1800s.[608] Congress recently released funds for manufacturers to develop and produce a new smallpox vaccine. It is likely to be made from a "diploid cell substrate" (human embryo) or from animal tissue cell cultures.[609-612]

Findings: During the 18th century, smallpox was common throughout Europe. In Sweden between 1774 and 1798, the annual incidence rate ranged from 3 to 10 cases per 1,000 people (about ½ percent to one percent of the population). In London between 1685 and 1801, the number of smallpox cases ranged from 3 to 24 per 1,000 (about ½ percent to nearly 2½ percent of the population). In Copenhagen between 1750 and 1800, smallpox cases ranged from 9 to 18 per 1,000 (about one percent to two percent of the population). Smallpox deaths during this period ranged from 1 per 5000 cases of the disease to 4 per 1000 cases (Figure 26).[613,614]

Smallpox had already stopped infecting people in more than 8 out of 10 countries throughout the world when the World Health Organization (WHO) launched a worldwide vaccination campaign against smallpox in 1967.[615] At that time, only 131,000 cases were reported.[616] Yet, authorities credit their global initiative with eliminating the disease. Some medical historians question the validity of this claim. Scarlet fever and the plague also infected millions of people. Vaccines were never developed for these diseases yet they disappeared as well.[617]

Figure 26:

Smallpox in 18th Century Europe: Annual Incidence Rates

Location	Years	Cases/1000	Population %
Sweden	1774-1798	3 to 10	.3 to 1.0
London	1685-1801	3 to 24	.3 to 2.4
Copenhagen	1750-1800	9 to 18	.9 to 1.8

Smallpox Deaths
Ranged from 1 death per 5000 cases (.0002 percent)
to 4 deaths per 1000 cases (.004 percent).

Copyright © 2002, NZM

Every year in Europe during the latter half of the 18th century, between 3 and 24 people per 1,000 contracted smallpox (less than ½ percent to almost 2½ percent of the population). Smallpox deaths ranged from 1 per 5000 cases to 4 per 1000 cases. Source: *Annals of Internal Medicine* (October 15, 1997).

Several reputable historians credit *multiple* public health activities—sanitation and nutrition reforms—with reducing the incidence and severity of the early problematic diseases, including smallpox, plague, dysentery, scarlet fever, typhoid, and cholera. During the late 18th and early 19th centuries, "the etiology of disease was largely unrecognized and the breeding places of disease were undiscovered."[618] With the advent of the industrial revolution, droves of people left the countryside to seek employment in the cities. Unsanitary and crowded living conditions contributed to the spread of disease.[619] Protective measures were inconsistently applied before health authorities coordinated community efforts to: 1) clean streets, backyards, and stables, 2) remove trash, construct sewage systems, and properly dispose of human waste, 3) drain swamps, marshes, and stagnant pools, 4) purify the water supply, 5) improve the roads so that food could be rapidly transported to the cities and distributed while still fresh and nutritious.[620,621]

Throughout the 1800s, several countries instituted compulsory vaccination laws. In 1807, vaccination was declared obligatory in Bavaria. In 1810, the shots were compulsory in Denmark.[622] England mandated smallpox vaccinations in 1853.[623] Prior to compulsory vaccine legislation, smallpox outbreaks were regional and self-limiting. The most severe epidemics occurred following mandatory shots. In England, from 1870 to 1872, after more than 15 years of forced immunizations—and a 98 percent vaccination rate[624]—the largest epidemic of smallpox ever recorded maimed and killed thousands of people. Most of the population had been vaccinated and re-vaccinated.[625] According to Dr. William Farr, Compiler of Statistics of the Registrar-General, London, "Smallpox attained its maximum mortality _after_ vaccination was introduced. The mean annual mortality to 10,000 population from 1850 to 1869 was at the rate of 2.04, whereas in 1871 the death rate was 10.24 and in 1872 the death rate was 8.33, and this after the most laudable efforts to extend vaccination by legislative enactments."[626]

Further corroboration of vaccine failures comes from Sir Thomas Chambers, a London health official: "Of the 155 persons admitted to the Smallpox Hospital in the Parish of St. James, Piccadilly, 145 had been vaccinated." Records from Marylevore Hospital indicate that 92 percent of the smallpox cases had been vaccinated. An official at Highgate Hospital confessed: "Of the 950 cases of smallpox [in 1871], 870 (92 percent) had been vaccinated." And records from the Hempstead Hospital show that up to May 13, 1884, out of 2,965 admissions for smallpox, 2,347 (79 percent) had been vaccinated.[627]

Figures were similar in many other countries where compulsory laws were established. For example, in 1870 and 1871, more than one million Germans contracted smallpox after Germany enforced mandatory shots; thousands died. Ninety-six percent of the victims were vaccinated.[628,629] According to the German Chancellor, "The hopes placed in the efficacy of the cowpox virus as a preventative of smallpox have proved entirely deceptive."[630] From 1887 to 1889, countless Italian citizens contracted smallpox after Italy enforced mandatory shots; thousands died.[631,632] According to Dr. Charles Rauta, Professor of Hygiene and Materia Medica at the University of Perguia, "Italy is one of the best vaccinated countries in the world... For 20 years before 1885, our nation was vaccinated in the proportion of 98.5 percent... The epidemics of smallpox that we have had [from 1887-1889] have been so frightful that nothing before the invention of vaccination could equal them."[633] From 1886 to 1908, hundreds of thousands of Japanese citizens contracted smallpox after Japan enforced mandatory shots every five years; thousands died.[634] And in 1918 and 1919, the worst epidemic of smallpox ever recorded in the Philippines occurred after the U.S. took control of the islands and enforced mandatory shots. The whole population was completely vaccinated; thousands died.[635,636] A 1920 Report

Figure 27:

Smallpox Deaths Tumbled
After People Refused the Vaccine

Ten-Year Period Ending:	% of Babies Vaccinated:	Smallpox Deaths (Annual Average):
1881	96.5	3708
1891	82.1	933
1901	67.9	437
1911	67.6	395
1921	42.3	12
1931	43.1	25
1941	39.9	1

Copyright © 2002, NZM

Source: Official statistics from England and Wales.

---

of the Philippine Health Service noted: "The 1918 epidemic looks prima facie as a flagrant failure of the classic immunization."[637] Clearly, there is an inverse correlation between the percentage of babies vaccinated and the number of smallpox deaths: the greater the number vaccinated, the greater the loss. Deaths from smallpox tumbled after people began refusing the shots (Figure 27).[638]

Several countries forbid vaccinations and/or enacted new legislation rescinding mandatory regulations. For example, according to the Secretary of the Governing Board in Dublin, Ireland, "Smallpox virus taken from the calf would communicate that disease to the human subject, and be thereby a fertile source of propagating the disease, and would, moreover, render the operator liable to prosecution under the Act prohibiting inoculation with smallpox."[639] In the late 1800s, Australia abolished compulsory vaccination and reported only three cases of smallpox in 15 years.[640]

Throughout the history of smallpox inoculations, intelligent people from all walks of life spoke out against the unscientific and perilous vaccine enterprise. For example, the great spiritual leader, Mahatma Gandhi, once stated: "I am, and have been for years, a confirmed anti-vaccinationist... I have not the least doubt in my mind that vaccination is a filthy process that is harmful in the end."[641]

Numerous doctors and health officials of the late 19th and early 20th centuries were vocal opponents of mandatory vaccines:[642-645]

"I have been a regular practitioner of medicine in Boston for 33 years. I have studied the question of vaccination conscientiously for 45 years. As for vaccination as a preventative disease, there is not a scrap of evidence in its favor. The injection of virus into the pure bloodstream of the people does not prevent smallpox; rather, it tends to increase its epidemics, and it makes the disease more deadly. Of this we have indisputable proof. In our country (U.S.) cancer mortality has increased from 9 per 100,000 to 80 per 100,000 or fully 900 percent increase within the past 50 years, and no conceivable thing could have caused this increase but the universal blood poisoning now existing."
—Dr. Charles E. Page, Boston practitioner

"Vaccination does not stay the spread of smallpox, nor even modify it in those who get it after vaccination. It does introduce in the system contamination and, therefore, contributes to the spread of tuberculosis, cancer, and even leprosy. It tends to make more virulent epidemics and to make them more extensive. It did just what inoculation did—cause the spread of disease."
—Dr. Walter M. James, Philadelphia practitioner

"Cancer was practically unknown until cowpox vaccination began to be introduced. I have had to do with 200 cases of cancer and I never saw a case of cancer in an unvaccinated person."
—Dr. W. B. Clark, New York practitioner

"I am convinced that some 80 percent of these cancer deaths are caused by the [smallpox] vaccinations they have undergone. These are well known to cause grave and permanent disease of the heart also."
—Dr. Herbert Snow, Surgeon, London Cancer Hospital

"Abolish vaccination, and you will cut the cancer death rate in half."
—Dr. F. P. Millard, Toronto practitioner

"Vaccines are principally responsible for the increase of those two really dangerous diseases, cancer and heart disease."
—Dr. Benchetrit, practitioner

"I am convinced that the increase of cancer is due to vaccination."
—Dr. Forbes Laurie, Medical Director of the Metropolitan Cancer Hospital, London

"It is my firm conviction that vaccination has been a curse instead of a blessing to the race. Every physician knows that cutaneous diseases (including cancer) have increased in frequency, severity, and variety to an alarming extent. To no medium of transmission is the widespread dissemination of this class of diseases so largely related as to vaccination."
—B. F. Cornell, M.D., practitioner

"I have removed cancers from vaccinated arms exactly where the poison was injected."
—Dr. E. J. Post, Michigan practitioner

"I have no hesitation in stating that in my judgment the most frequent disposing condition for cancerous development is infused into the blood by vaccination and re-vaccination."
—Dr. Dennis Turnbull, 30 year cancer researcher

"Never in the history of medicine has there been produced so false a theory, and such fraudulent assumptions, such disastrous and damning results as have followed the practice of vaccination; it is the ultma thule (extremity) of learned quackery, and lacks, and has ever lacked, the faintest shadow of a scientific basis. The fears of the people have been played upon as to the dangers of smallpox, and the promise of sure prevention by vaccination, until nearly the whole civilized world has become physically corrupted by its practice."
—Dr. E. Ripley, Connecticut practitioner

"I now have very little faith in vaccination, even as to modifying the disease, and none at all as a protective in virulent epidemics. Personally, I contracted smallpox less than six months after a most severe vaccination."
—Dr. R. Hall Bakewell, Vaccinator General of Trinidad

"Vaccination is the infusion of contaminating elements into the system, and after such contamination you can never be sure of regaining the former purity of the body. Consumption (tuberculosis) follows in the wake of vaccination just as surely as effect follows cause."
—Dr. Alexander Wilder, professor of pathology, U.S. Medical College of New York

"In looking over the history of vaccination for smallpox, I am amazed to learn of the terrible deaths from vaccination which necessitated amputation of arms and legs and caused tetanus, foot-and-mouth disease, septicemia (blood poisoning), and cerebro-spinal meningitis."
—Dr. R. C. Carter, practitioner

Several studies and official declarations confirm that smallpox vaccines were dangerous and ineffective. For example, in 1915 the United States Department of Agriculture traced several epidemics of foot-and-mouth disease to the smallpox vaccine.[646,647] In July 1926, the *Journal of the American Medical Association* found correlations between smallpox vaccinations and neurological disorders. The authors noted: "In regions in which there is no organized vaccination of the population, general paralysis is rare. In patients with general paralysis...vaccination scars were always present."[648] In September 1926, *Lancet* published data confirming encephalomyelitis following smallpox vaccinations. The authors declared: "There can be no doubt that vaccination was a definite causal factor."[649] In October 1926, *Lancet* again reported on numerous cases of encephalitis following smallpox vaccinations. Many of the victims died. The authors concluded: "Vaccination was a definite causal factor and no chance coincidence."[650] And in 1928, the *British Medical Journal* confessed that people vaccinated against smallpox were five times more likely to die from the disease than those who were not vaccinated.[651,652]

During the late 1950s and 1960s, several medical and scientific publications, including the *British Medical Journal* and *Pediatrics,* documented numerous cases of post-vaccinal encephalomyeltis following smallpox vaccination. Neurological reactions ranged from encephalitis to epilepsy, polyneuritis, multiple sclerosis, and death. In some regions of the world, one of every 63 people vaccinated was damaged by the shot.[653-659]

In 1987, the *New England Journal of Medicine* reported on a military recruit who contracted AIDS after being vaccinated against smallpox. Doctors who reviewed the case wrote: "Primary smallpox immunization of persons with subclinical HIV disease poses a risk of vaccine-induced disease [and] multiple immunizations may accelerate the progress of HIV disease. This case raises concern about the ultimate safety of vaccinia-based vaccine in developing countries where HIV infection is increasing."[660]

Two months later, the *London Times* published a compelling report indicating "the AIDS epidemic may have been triggered by the mass vaccination campaign" against smallpox.[661] The *Times* exposé was written in response to a tip from an advisor to the World Health Organization who was assigned by WHO to investigate the suspicion that its ambitious vaccination program in Africa had caused the AIDS epidemic. The WHO advisor did his study, concluded that the smallpox vaccine was a trigger for AIDS, and filed his report with WHO. When the report was buried, he contacted the *Times.*[662]

The greatest concentration of AIDS coincided with regions where the smallpox vaccination program was most intense—Zaire, Zambia, Tanzania, Uganda, Malawi, Ruanda, and Burundi. Brazil was the only South American country included in the vaccination campaign, and it had the highest incidence of AIDS on that continent. Haiti also had a high incidence of the disease. Several thousand Haitians were on a United Nations mission in Central Africa when WHO conducted its mass vaccination campaign; they received smallpox inoculations.[663,664]

The WHO advisor told the *Times,* "I thought it was just a coincidence until we studied the latest findings about the reactions which can be caused by vaccinia. Now I believe the smallpox vaccination theory is the explanation of AIDS."[665] Dr. Robert Gallo, renowned authority on AIDS, also accepts the possibility: "I have been saying for some years that the use of live vaccines such as that used for smallpox can activate a dormant infection such as HIV."[666] This has led some experts to fear that an attempt to control one disease, smallpox, transformed another disease, AIDS, "from a minor endemic illness of the Third World into the current pandemic."[667]

On September 11, 2001, 19 terrorists hijacked four American commercial jets and flew them into occupied buildings killing approximately 3,000 people. A few weeks later, bioterrorists mailed deadly anthrax to U.S. politicians and media personnel. Hundreds of people were exposed to the germ; several died.[668-670] These actions raised immediate concerns regarding how to protect innocent people from biological threats. However, even though government health officials have identified several diseases that would wreak havoc if terrorists successfully circulated the germs, including botulism, ebola, tularemia, and plague,[671] authorities chose to concentrate their resources on developing a "new and improved" smallpox vaccine.

In June of 2001, just three months prior to the terrorist attack, a team of bioterrorism specialists, led by the Johns Hopkins University Center for Civilian Biodefense Studies, conducted an exercise code-named Dark Winter that simulated an outbreak of smallpox in the United States. Within two months after the hypothetical epidemic started, three million people were infected. Dark Winter ended with the collapse of interstate commerce, crowds rioting in the streets, and the nation moving toward martial law.[672] However, like any theoretical exercise, conclusions are predicated on the underlying assumptions. One key assumption was that each person with smallpox would infect at least 10 other people and that those 10 people would each infect at least 10 more people and so on.[673] But a recent CDC study published in *Emerging Infectious Diseases* regards those infection rates as grossly unrealistic. The authors of the CDC study looked at data from numerous smallpox outbreaks and reported that on average less than one person was infected per infectious person. In all outbreaks, some infected persons did not transmit a case of smallpox to another person. The researchers even cited evidence of 12 unvaccinated persons who had face-to-face contact with an infected person; none of the 12 became ill with clinical cases of smallpox. The CDC researchers concluded "the probability that the average transmission rate will be greater than two cannot be demonstrated..."[674,675] Thus, the Dark Winter simulation was seriously flawed. Nevertheless, team leaders urged authorities to support an immediate increase in the production and delivery of smallpox vaccine.[676]

Researchers have no evidence that a new smallpox vaccine will cause fewer adverse reactions than the old vaccine. According to Franklin Top, a biotechnology expert who previously served as the commander of the Walter Reed Army Institute of Research, reactogenicity "is going to be a problem."[677] According to Dr. Frank Fenner, one of the world's leading authorities on smallpox, "the risk of vaccination with ordinary smallpox vaccine [in countries with high levels of HIV] would be dangerous."[678] He does not believe that reintroducing vaccination will provide a simple solution. Dr. Mark Buller, a virologist who is investigating safer smallpox treatments at St. Louis University is even more candid: "I would not even consider having my family vaccinated. I'm more likely to be hit riding my bike to work than to be hit by a smallpox episode in my own life."[679] And scientists may never be able to create a vaccine that can protect against mutated strains of the virus. Dozens of strains already exist.[680] New permutations of the variola microbe could be developed by bioterrorists rendering a new vaccine worthless, thus subjecting recipients of the shot to the inherent risk of serious adverse reactions without the expected benefit.[681]

On October 23, 2001, the CDC unveiled newly proposed legislation—_The Model State Emergency Health Powers Act_[682] —giving public health officials and state governors the authority to arrest, vaccinate, medicate, and quarantine anyone they deem either unprotected from, or a threat to spread, infectious disease.[683] Local police and the U.S. military, by way of the National Guard, would enforce the law.[684,685] Previous laws permitting medical, religious, or philosophical exemptions would be repealed.[686]

The proposed bill also threatens to seize private property for use by the state, to control access to communications, and to limit legal recourse. In fact, once a "public health emergency" is declared, the U.S. Constitution, Bill of Rights, and civil liberties will be suspended. Furthermore, this "model legislation" exempts the State, the police, the militia, and public health authorities from any liability due to their actions. If an individual opposes vaccines, is force-inoculated and dies, the perpetrators cannot be prosecuted.[687]

Special Reports:
Booklets containing comprehensive data on the individual vaccines are available. For more information, visit:
http://thinktwice.com/booklets.htm

FLU

Influenza, or the flu, is a contagious respiratory infection caused by a virus. It usually strikes during winter. Symptoms include fever, chills, runny nose, sore throat, cough, headache, muscle aches, fatigue, and decreased appetite. Conditions usually improve in two to three days. Treatment mainly consists of allowing the disease to run its course. Antibiotics will not subdue the flu virus. Bed rest and drinking lots of fluids are often recommended.

The flu can lead to complications, such as pneumonia, in high risk groups—mainly the elderly and people with heart, lung, or kidney dysfunctions, diabetes, anemia, or compromised immune systems. In some circumstances, severe complications in high risk groups can lead to death.

There are three main types of flu virus. Each type can mutate, or change, from year to year. This makes it difficult to develop immunity to the disease.[688] Thus, every year health officials produce a new flu vaccine containing the three types of flu virus. For example, the influenza vaccine prepared for the 1999-2000 season included Sydney, Beijing, and Shangdong-like disease antigens.[689] The 2000-2001 flu vaccine contained Moscow, Beijing, and New Caledonia-like strains of the virus.[690]

Findings: To produce a flu vaccine, chick embryos are inoculated with influenza viruses. This mixture is cultivated for several weeks. Each flu strain is then inactivated with formaldehyde and preserved with thimerosal, a mercury derivative.[691,692] The three viral strains are then blended into a single vaccine, licensed by the FDA and distributed by vaccine manufacturers. Scientific control-group testing for safety and efficacy is not required.[693]

Common reactions to the flu shot include flu-like symptoms which can last several days: fever, chills, headache, muscle aches, and fatigue.[694,695] Doctors claim that it's not possible to contract the flu from the flu vaccine. But this contradicts the real-life experiences of many people. Besides, vaccines are designed to stimulate the immune system by mimicking disease.

Serious reactions to the flu vaccine include life-threatening allergies to vaccine components, and Guillain-Barré syndrome (GBS), a severe paralytic disease.[696-699] GBS can occur several weeks following a flu vaccine and is fatal in about one of every 20 victims.[700] In addition to GBS, numerous studies have investigated and/or documented other serious adverse reactions to the flu vaccine, including encephalopathy, brain stem encephalitis, polyneuritis, arthritis, and thrombocytopenia (a serious blood disorder).[701-736]

The _Thinktwice Global Vaccine Institute_ receives unsolicited reports of adverse reactions to the flu vaccine:

"I received a flu shot in November, and in January I started to get a body rash. I am achy in my (vaccine) arm and neck. I believe the shot may be responsible for my misery."

"My wife was diagnosed with subcutaneous T-cell lymphoma after receiving a flu shot."

"I have a friend who received a flu vaccine on Monday and by Tuesday was very sick. After many tests the doctors said it was not a reaction to the flu shot. Their diagnosis was 'reactivated mono' —despite the fact that she never had mono. I have heard many people swear that they'll never get another flu vaccine. Now I understand."

"The sister of an acquaintance died suddenly two nights ago. She was in her 40s and otherwise healthy. She got a flu shot that day, came home complaining about not feeling well, and died that night. She died at home, rather suddenly, without warning. Do you know if this is an unusual coincidence or a recurring pattern?"

"I need information to heal a friend who received the flu shot five weeks ago and is having extreme pain in the arms, legs, and neck, with paralyzation. The doctors won't help."

"My grandmother was given a flu injection and immediately contracted the worst case of pneumonia she had ever had. She was so sick that she nearly died. Now she has severe joint pain that has lasted ever since her shot."

"My husband's aunt, who was very healthy before she got a flu shot, became ill after the shot for about four weeks, never improving, until she died."

"Two weeks ago one of our patients died three days after her flu vaccine. The day after her shot, her daughter came into our clinic to apologize that her mother couldn't keep her appointment with us, explaining that she had a bad reaction to her flu shot. That was on a Friday. The following Monday we were reading the lovely lady's obituary. Her death was not reported as a reaction to the flu shot."[737]

Precise flu vaccine efficacy rates are difficult to ascertain and unreliable because flu strains change all the time. According to the CDC, "Overall vaccine effectiveness varies from year to year, depending upon the degree of similarity between the influenza virus strains included in the vaccine and the strain or strains that circulate during the influenza season."[738] Furthermore, although many doctors and other health authorities contend that the flu vaccine cannot cause the flu, the CDC acknowledges that "people who have received [the flu] vaccine may indeed have an influenza infection."[739]

To understand why flu vaccines are so problematic, it is important to know how authorities try to control this unpredictable virus. Production of each new flu vaccine, to be distributed in fall, usually begins in January. Therefore, officials must guess one year in advance which mutated strains of the flu virus will circulate throughout society.[740] If they guess right, the vaccine is thought to be about 35 percent effective at temporarily preventing that year's flu in the elderly.[741,742] If they guess wrong, as often occurs, or the circulating strains mutate again between January and the end of the year, which is likely, the vaccine may be worthless.[743,744] For example, in 1994 flu "experts" predicted that the Shangdong, Texas, and Panama strains would be prevalent that year, thus millions of people received flu shots containing these strains. However, when winter arrived, the Johannesburg and Beijing strains were circulating. In 1995, health officials modified their predictions and created a flu vaccine that contained the Texas, Johannesburg, and Beijing strains. Again, millions of people were vaccinated. However, when winter arrived, the Wuhan strain predominated.[745] During the 1997-1998 flu season, officials once more had to admit that "the flu shot did not make a dent in flu cases because the strains included in the vaccine did not match the strains that actually circulated that year."[746] The vaccine was zero percent effective (Figure 28).

More recently, the 2003-2004 flu vaccine was designed to protect against the Panama strain. However, the Fujian strain dominated that year's flu season. A CDC study concluded that the vaccine had "no or low effectiveness."[747] In fact, authorities knew several months in advance that the Fujian strain was the most likely to circulate that year, and that their "Panama" flu shot would not protect against it, yet they frightened the public by predicting a deadly flu season, then exploited the masses with their worthless vaccine.[748]

Even when there is a good match between the viral strains in a flu vaccine and that year's circulating flu virus, immunity from the shot is short-lived because antibody levels begin to decline within months, and are often low one year after vaccination.[749] Permanent immunity to a particular strain of flu is only possible by contracting the disease naturally. Further evidence of poor flu vaccine efficacy rates in the elderly may be found in other studies.[750-752] For example, in one influenza outbreak in a Minnesota nursing home, 95 percent of the residents, and 72 percent of the staff members with direct patient contact had been vaccinated 4-8 weeks prior to the outbreak.

Figure 28:

Flu Vaccine Efficacy in the Elderly

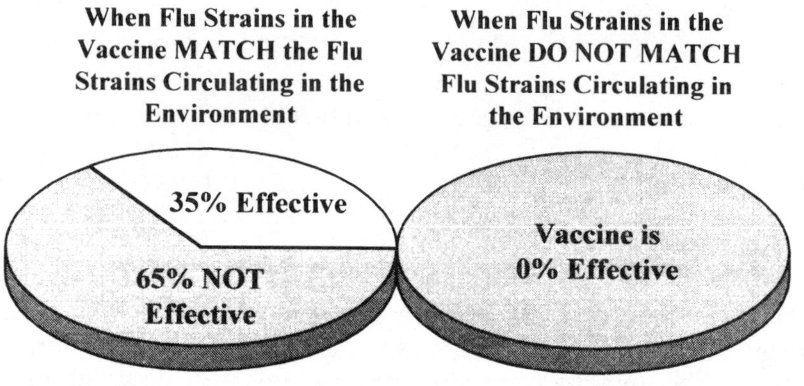

When Flu Strains in the Vaccine MATCH the Flu Strains Circulating in the Environment

When Flu Strains in the Vaccine DO NOT MATCH Flu Strains Circulating in the Environment

35% Effective

65% NOT Effective

Vaccine is 0% Effective

Copyright © 2002, Neil Z. Miller

Every year, health officials must guess which strains of the flu will circulate throughout society. When they guess right, and their vaccine contains flu strains matching that year's circulating flu, the shot is about 35% effective in preventing that year's flu in the elderly. When they guess wrong, the vaccine offers NO protection against the flu. Source: Several CDC *MMWRs*.

Authorities were baffled when they learned that the viral strain isolated from the outbreak was "antigenically identical" to the one contained in the vaccine. In other words, the vaccine was a "perfect" match for that year's circulating flu virus, yet it was a complete failure. Authors of the study concluded that "despite widespread vaccination...influenza outbreaks continue to occur..."[753]

Other respiratory ailments, intestinal disorders and ear infections caused by bacteria, disease conditions caused by flu viruses not included in the vaccine, or by microorganisms associated with different diseases, such as colds, will not be alleviated by getting an annual flu shot. Each flu vaccine is only designed to protect against the three viral strains included in that year's flu vaccine.

In June 2003, FluMist, a flu vaccine squirted up the nose, was approved for people ages 5 to 49 years—even though the young and elderly are at greatest risk. Annual sales of up to $1 billion are expected.[754] Beginning September 2004, the CDC recommends the needle-driven flu shot for all infants 6 months of age or older.[755]

In past years, the CDC strongly encouraged the elderly to receive annual flu shots. Recently, the Advisory Committee on Immunization

Figure 29:

Annual Flu Shots:
Do Doctors and Nurses Get Them?

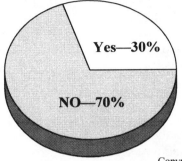

Copyright © 2002, Neil Z. Miller

Although doctors want *you* to receive an annual flu shot, surveys show that doctors and nurses are among the *least* likely to be vaccinated. In fact, about 70 percent of doctors and nurses do NOT get annual flu shots. Source: *Associated Press* (October 9, 1997).

Practices (ACIP) "recommended" that all nursing home residents and staff members receive annual flu vaccinations.[756] The ACIP's recommendations generally result in medical coercion and compulsory immunizations. For example, one health worker reported: "The hospital where I have worked for the past 15 years is now forcing all employees to take an influenza vaccine. We have no choice but to take the shot or be disallowed to work. I strongly disagree with this issue. My rights and freedoms are being trampled on."[757]

Even though health care workers are being forced to receive annual flu vaccinations or lose their jobs, studies have shown that following mass vaccinations of nursing home residents and staff members, everyone still remains at risk of contracting the disease.[758] The elderly do not like being forced-injected either. But this is exactly what authorities are requiring. Many long-term nursing home residents must now choose between the flu vaccine and finding a new place to live and be cared for. Yet in one recent survey, nearly 4 million elderly people refused *free* influenza shots.[759] And although doctors want *you* to receive an annual flu vaccination, surveys show that doctors and nurses are among the *least* likely to be vaccinated. In fact, more than two-thirds (about 70 percent) of doctors and nurses do NOT get annual flu shots (Figure 29).[760]

MULTIPLE VACCINES

The current schedule of "recommended" vaccines is so crowded that doctors are administering several shots during a single office visit, often with disastrous results. This section contains unsolicited reports of adverse reactions following the administration of several vaccines simultaneously. These reports are typical of the daily emails received by the *Thinktwice Global Vaccine Institute*.

"My son received his DTaP shot and Prevnar. The following morning he had seven seizures. He would go ghost-white and throw out his arms. They would be rigid and jerking. He stared straight ahead and didn't breathe. He used to say mama and dada [before the shots]. Now he only babbles. He is far behind in all areas tested."

"My son has had five seizures since his last shots (DTaP, Hib and MMR). He was sick at the time. They gave him his shots anyway, telling me it didn't matter. What can I do?"

"After my son received his DPT, Hib, polio, and hepatitis B shots, he developed a persistent cough, then pneumonia and an ear infection. This 'ear infection' has lasted almost six weeks."

"My daughter was fine until she had her second Hib and DT vaccines. She became ill after this and was unable to grasp anything. She went from a very vocal, social five-month-old to a withdrawn silent seven-month-old who failed her checkup on all counts."

"I experienced a very acute reaction to several vaccines I received (MMR, hepatitis A, hepatitis B, and yellow fever) prior to leaving the country. I still suffer every day from these ill effects: fatigue, joint pain, restlessness, and cognitive dysfunction."

"After my baby had her six-month shots (DTaP, oral polio, and Hib) she had what the emergency room doctor considered a febrile seizure. She was fine until then. Three days later the doctor said she had streptococcal pneumonia. When she is not sleeping, she wriggles and cries like she is in pain."

"My son was born premature, just 3lbs, 3oz at birth. At his two-month check the nurse said he need his shots. I argued with her but she gave him four shots. I will never forget the scream he let out. Less than 24 hours later he died—and I was accused of his death!"

"My normal, healthy 12-month-old daughter was vaccinated with hepatitis B, polio, and varicella. The next day she began to vomit and did not stop for two hours. She became completely lethargic and ended up in the emergency room with IV fluid pumping through her to keep her alive. All the medical staff told me this could not be a reaction to her vaccinations. What do you think?"[761]

Long-Term Effects

Few serious attempts have been made to discover the long-term effects of injecting foreign proteins and toxic substances into the healthy bodies of innocent infants. In fact, research focusing on possible correlations between vaccines, autoimmune diseases, and neurologically-based disorders (i.e., multiple sclerosis, cerebral palsy, Guillain-Barré syndrome, cancer, and AIDS) is just beginning. For example, one medical researcher, Dr. Richard Moskowitz, concluded that the unnatural process of vaccination can lead to slow viruses developing in the body. These may bring about the "far less curable chronic diseases of the present."[762] He also noted that "these illnesses may be considerably more serious than the original disease, involving deeper structures [and] more vital organs."[763] Other researchers have identified a "lowering of the body's resistance resulting from vaccinations." They warn us about the "probability of widespread and unrecognized vaccine-induced immune system malfunction." They also note that this effect is often delayed, indirect, and masked, its true nature seldom recognized.[764]

The Immune System: Several researchers have noted that vaccines merely "trick" the body into focusing on only one aspect (antibody production) of the many complex and integrated strategies normally available to the immune system. Diseases contracted naturally are filtered through a series of immune system defenses. But when the vaccine virus is injected directly into the child's bloodstream, it gains access to all of the major tissues and organs of the body *without the body's normal advantage of a total immune response.*[765] Antibodies (T-lymphocytes) that do respond to the invading vaccine germs become committed to those germs and are unable to react to other challenges to the health of the child.[766,767] Research indicates that the immature immune system of a baby is stimulated, strengthened, and matured by responding to *natural* challenges. When the infant gains exposure to viral and bacterial microorganisms *in the environment*, normal development of the immune system is likely to occur. However, if the immature immune system is forced to respond to a barrage of vaccinations injected directly into the body, bypassing outer immune system defenses, inner immune system protective maneuvers may be overwhelmed. When natural immunity is curtailed and the immune system compelled to operate in unnatural ways, questions arise regarding its ability to protect the child throughout life.[768]

The immune system is designed to help the organism discriminate "self" from everything else that is foreign and potentially dangerous to the self. Under natural conditions, enemy germs are attacked and rendered benign by the immune system. But alien viruses injected into the body fuse with healthy cells, and continue to replicate along with those cells.[769] This is likely to confuse the immune system, which can no longer differentiate between harmful and harmless conditions within the body. Under these circumstances, the immune system is likely to either invade its own cells (cancer), or ignore danger signs altogether, leaving the organism vulnerable to any number of autoimmune diseases.[770]

Autopsies were performed comparing the thymus glands (responsible for the production of protective T-cells) of adults in poorly vaccinated countries versus adults in the United States. Researchers found that in the U.S., thymus glands begin to atrophy following puberty. Thymus gland deterioration was found to be minimal in adults from the poorly vaccinated countries. Thymus gland abnormalities are associated with a variety of autoimmune and tumor producing diseases (e.g., many different types of cancer, leukemia, lupus erythematosus, and rheumatoid arthritis). Some researchers blame this situation on the widespread, mandatory childhood vaccination programs.[771]

Genetic Mutations: The polio vaccine contains monkey kidney cell culture and calf serum. Other vaccines are prepared in chick embryo. Monkey kidney, calf serum, and chick embryo are foreign proteins—biological matter composed of animal cells. Because they are injected directly into the bloodstream, they are able to change our genetic structure.[772,773]

Viruses (and viral vaccines) are agents for the transfer of genetic imprints from one host to another. Because they contain pure genetic material (DNA and RNA) from a foreign organism, once injected into a human recipient, the new genetic material is incorporated into the invaded cells.[774] There is a lot of literature confirming the action of viruses in bringing about genetic changes in unrelated organisms.[775,776] As early as the 1950s, Barbara McClintock, an American geneticist, described mobile genetic elements—"jumping genes."[777] In the 1960s, Joshua Lederberg, from the Department of Genetics, Stanford University, notified the scientific world that "live viruses are...genetic messages used for the purpose of programming human cells." He was also notably explicit when he said that "we already practice biological engineering on a rather large scale by use of live viruses in mass immunization campaigns."[778]

No one knows the long-term effects of tampering with the genetic codes and delicate structure of the human organism. However, the physical invasion of the human body by foreign genetic material may have the immediate effect of permanently weakening the immune system, setting in motion a new era of autoimmune diseases.[779] For example, research indicates that psychotic disorders may be caused by viral infections.[780-782] The incidence of schizophrenia is on the rise compared to earlier times,[783] and studies indicate that about one-third of all cases are autoimmune in nature.[784] Some authorities implicate the childhood vaccine programs.[785]

Developmental Disabilities: According to the medical historian, Harris L. Coulter, Ph.D., "the family and society are both victims of vaccination programs forced on them by state legislatures that are entirely too responsive to medical opinion and medical organizations." The entire postwar American generation is suffering from what he calls "post-encephalitic syndrome"—the name he gives to define a variety of vaccine-induced disabilities.[786] To support his assertions, Coulter presented evidence showing that the long-term effects of vaccinations may be more pervasive than suspected. However, disabilities caused by the vaccines are often "disguised" under different names: autism, dyslexia, learning disability, epilepsy, mental retardation, hyperactivity, and minimal brain dysfunction, to name a few. Juvenile delinquency, an unprecedented rise in violent crime, drug abuse, and the collapse of the American school system unable to contend with the estimated 20 to 25 percent of students mentally and emotionally deficient, represent other conditions that may be attributed to the vaccines.[787]

The developmental disabilities and other conditions noted above are frequently caused by encephalitis, or inflammation of the brain. Medical practitioners know that encephalitis can be caused by a severe injury to the head, a severe burn, from an infectious disease, *or from the vaccines against these diseases*—post-vaccinal encephalitis.[788] *The principal cause of encephalitis in the United States today, and in other industrialized countries, is childhood vaccination programs.*[789] The symptoms of post-vaccinal encephalitis are identical to the symptoms of encephalitis arising from any other cause.[790] Since any segment of the nervous system may be affected, every possible physical, intellectual, and personality deviation, and combinations of them, are possible.[791,792]

Autopsies after post-vaccinal encephalitis show a loss and destruction of myelin on the brainstem and spinal cord. Myelin covers and protects the nerves much like the insulation on an electric wire. Without myelin, nerve impulses are short-circuited and the nervous system remains undeveloped and immature.[793]

An overt reaction to the vaccine is not required to confirm that damage to the central nervous system was caused by post-vaccinal encephalitis. In fact, there is no correlation between the degree of cerebral damage that may later ensue and the severity of the condition that lead to encephalitis in the first place.[794-798] In other words, subtle and often overlooked reactions to the vaccine (i.e., a slight fever, fussiness, drowsiness) can be, and often is, a case of encephalitis which is capable of causing severe neurological complications months or even years later.[799]

Now let's look at some of the specific disabilities that may be attributed to post-vaccinal encephalitis:

Autism: In 1943, the well known child psychiatrist, Leo Kanner, announced his discovery of eleven cases of a new mental disorder. He noted that "the condition differs markedly and uniquely from anything reported so far..."[800] This condition soon became known as autism. (Autism is a type of brain damage. Children with this disorder are frequently retarded, mute, and unresponsive to human contact.) These first cases of autism in the United States occurred at a time when the pertussis vaccine was becoming increasingly available. By the 1950s and 1960s, parents from all over the country were seeking help for their autistic children. The growing numbers of children suffering from this new illness directly coincided with the growing popularity of the mandated vaccination programs during these same years. By the late 1980s, over 4500 new cases of autism were occurring every year in the U.S. alone.[801]

The same correlations between autism and childhood vaccination programs may be found in other countries as well. When the United States ended the war and occupied Japan, a mandatory vaccination program was established. The first autistic Japanese child was born in 1945.[802] Today, hundreds of new cases of autism are diagnosed in Japanese children every year.[803] Europe received the pertussis vaccine in the 1950s; the first cases of autism began to appear there in the same decade. In England the pertussis vaccine wasn't promoted on a large scale until the late 1950s. Shortly thereafter, in 1962, the National Society for Autistic Children in Britain was established.[804]

When the first cases of autism began to appear, researchers were puzzled by the high incidence of autistic children being born into well-educated families. Over 90 percent of the parents were high school graduates. Nearly three-fourths of the fathers and one-half of the mothers had graduated from college. Many had professional careers. Thus, scientists tried to link autism to genetic factors in upper class populations.[805] Meanwhile, psychiatrists, unaware of the neurological basis of the illness, sought psychological explanations. Mothers were blamed for restrained emotions.[806,807]

In the 1970s, socioeconomic disparities began to disappear.[808] Once again this puzzled the researchers. Many simply concluded that earlier studies were flawed. But there is an explanation. When the pertussis vaccine was initially introduced, only the rich and educated parents who sought the very best for their children, and who could afford a private doctor, were in a position to request the newest medical advances. Free vaccinations at public health clinics didn't yet exist. Compulsory vaccination programs were still on the horizon. But as vaccine programs grew, parents from across the socioeconomic spectrum gained equal access to them. Thus, autistic children were soon being discovered within every kind of family, and in dreadfully greater numbers than ever before imagined.[809]

In the 1980s and 1990s, cases of autism soared once again. For example, California experienced a 273 percent increase since 1988.[810] The U.S. Department of Education showed a 556 percent increase from 1991 to 1997.[811] Today, in some parts of the country, 1 of every 400 children is autistic. Many researchers implicate the MMR vaccine—introduced and aggressively marketed during this period.[812]

In 1998, *Lancet* published a landmark study by Dr. Andrew Wakefield linking the onset of autistic symptoms to the MMR vaccine.[813] Recent studies by Dr. F. Edward Yazbak also show a significant correlation between MMR and autism, especially when the shot is delivered around pregnancy.[814-816] (These studies and many others are thoroughly reviewed in *Vaccines, Autism and Childhood Disorders: A Parent's Guide to MMR*.)[817] Eventually, on April 6, 2000, Congress gathered several experts, as well as parents of MMR-damaged children, to study the apparent connection between MMR and autism. This triple vaccine was clearly implicated as a causative factor.[818] (The testimony can be read at: www.thinktwice.com) A few months later, Dr. Walter Schilling published the results of his independent research suggesting that children who receive all of the recommended vaccines are "approximately 14 times more likely to become learning disabled and eight times more likely to become autistic" when compared to children who are never vaccinated.[819]

The _Thinktwice Global Vaccine Institute_ receives numerous reports of an MMR-autism link. Here are a few of these reports:

"When our beautiful, healthy, only son was 15 months old, he was given his routine MMR vaccine. Within four days he was at death's door with meningitis. He could no longer speak, walk, eat, or see. His behavior could best be described as autistic."

"Prior to my son's MMR vaccine he said loads of words. Now he has very little speech and is moderately autistic. If I could turn back the clock, I would, but now I have to live with the knowledge that we did not protect him; we let them damage him beyond repair."

"My 10-year-old son was healthy until nine days after his MMR vaccine at age 16 months. He had two febrile seizures and a measles rash, then lost his few words of speech over the next week."

"Exactly 14 days after my son's MMR vaccination, he had measles and mumps-type reactions. He has now been diagnosed as autistic. He also has leaky gut syndrome and asthma. My son was in PERFECT health up until the day of his reaction. He lost all powers of speech on that day and has never regained them."

"After my son's MMR shot at 12 months, his development and personality changed. He would stare off and not notice anything, not even the waving of my hand in front of his face. His personality became nothing—he lost all words and still has none. It is so hard to see my only son lose his personality and life to a shot."[820]

Hyperactivity/Minimal Brain Dysfunction: In the 1950s, another disorder rapidly spread among school children and gained prominence in the medical science and health literature: hyperactivity (attention-deficit hyperactivity disorder—ADHD). In 1963, the U.S. Public Health Service listed dozens of symptoms associated with hyperactivity and officially changed the name to "minimal brain dysfunction" (MBD). By the 1970s, some leading authorities noted that this disorder appeared to lie at the root of nearly every type of childhood behavior problem, and had become the most commonly diagnosed illness among child guidance counselors.[821] In 1988, the _Journal of the American Medical Association_ acknowledged that minimal brain damage had become the leading disability reported by elementary schools, and "one of the most common referral problems to child psychiatry outpatient clinics."[822] In some school districts, up to 13 percent of the children are now enrolled in "special education classes."[823] But minimally brain damaged children often go undetected, and some researchers believe that the actual figures for children with this disorder are closer to 15 to 20 percent.[824]

Although many children are not diagnosed as learning disabled or minimally brain damaged, teachers complain that nearly all of their students are cognitively inferior and have shorter attention spans when compared to kids they taught in the 1960s.[825] One instructor notes that when she gives directions many forget them almost immediately, even after several repetitions. "They look around, fidget, and doodle."[826] Another teacher laments that "kids' brains must be different these days."[827] In fact, beginning in 1964 the average SAT verbal and math scores have continued to steadily decline.[828] In an attempt to appease school administrators, who are often blamed for declining scores, and to safeguard the truth, test-makers have been "dumbing down" their tests since the 1960s. Our children today are taking tests much more simple than those given decades ago.[829]

Like autism, minimal brain dysfunction was initially thought to have psychological origins. But these children usually exhibit symptoms associated with neurological damage: seizure disorders, tics, tremors, infantile spasms, EEG abnormalities, motor impairments, poor visual-motor coordination, and cranial nerve palsies (capable of causing visual defects, eye disturbances, and hearing and speech impediments).[830] A few brief examples of the neurological basis for minimal brain dysfunction are given below:

- ► Harold reacted to his 2nd DPT shot with high-pitched screaming (the "cri encephalique"). Harold is now blind.[831]
- ► Kate was four months old when she received the DPT shot. Within 72 hours she was shrieking in pain. Today she continues to have seizures and cannot speak.[832]
- ► Wesley reacted to his 2nd DPT shot with glazed eyes and seizures. Today he continues to have up to 30 seizures daily, and has been diagnosed as permanently brain damaged.[833]
- ► Judy had her first grand mal seizure seven days after her 2nd DPT shot. Today she has a very low attention span and tends to reverse letters and write things backwards.[834]
- ► Ralph reacted to his first three DPT shots with persistent crying and a 104 degree fever. Today he has visual perception problems and cannot read or write correctly.[835]
- ► On the fourth day after 6-year-old Cassidy received her measles shot, she turned deathly ill and collapsed following a seizure. Today she is developmentally delayed.[836]

Violent Crime: A disproportionate amount of violent crime is committed by individuals with neurological damage.[837] For example, as early as the 1920s researchers were aware that children who had "recovered" from encephalitis were more likely to engage in abusive, cruel, and destructive behavior. Such children were called "apaches."[838,839] Today we call these children juvenile delinquents (suffering from hyperactivity or conduct disorder), but their numbers are now of epidemic proportions and their crimes are more violent.[840] Dyslexia and other learning disabilities have been found in nearly 90 percent of delinquents.[841] Delinquent children with these disorders are often reclassified as sociopaths upon reaching adulthood.[842]

Studies confirm that children with neurologically based disorders often engage in violent criminal behavior as adolescents and adults. In one study, hyperactive children were twenty times more likely than the rest of the population to end up in a reform school.[843] In another study, half of the incarcerated delinquents had an IQ below 85.[844] A report in the _Journal of the American Medical Association_ acknowledged that a disproportionate number of felons suffered from hyperactivity (ADHD) during their earlier years.[845]

Epilepsy and seizure disorders frequently occur following cases of post-vaccinal encephalitis. Studies indicate that epileptics find it significantly more difficult to control their impulses and aggressiveness.[846] In one study, the prevalence of prisoners with a history of seizures was found to be nearly ten times greater than the general population.[847] In another study of 321 mostly white, middle-class, extremely violent individuals, more than 90 percent showed evidence of brain damage, including a medical history implicating epilepsy.[848]

Drug Abuse: Psychiatrists and pediatricians prescribe a variety of drugs to young children to control hyperactivity and MBD. In one study, it was estimated that six percent of U.S. children rely on these compounds to render them "manageable." In some regions, where doctors "specialize" in these disorders, the percentage is much greater.[849] Many of these drugs have adverse side effects that are considered by some researchers to be worse than the original symptoms. These new symptoms are sometimes irreversible.[850]

Many people who have studied the above problems believe that the medical abuse of drugs in school children predisposes them to abuse "street drugs" later in life.[851] Adolescents suffering from minimal brain dysfunction are at risk for engaging in unusually early smoking, drinking, and substance abuse.[852] Adults with this disorder are also notably susceptible to alcoholism and the misuse of drugs.[853]

Additional Information

In 1986, Congress passed the *National Childhood Vaccine Injury Act.* This federal law contains two main elements: safety provisions, and a no-fault federal compensation program. The safety reform portion of the law requires doctors to: a) provide parents with information about childhood diseases and vaccines *prior* to vaccination; b) report vaccine reactions to federal health officials; c) record vaccine reactions in an individual's permanent record; and d) keep a record of the date that each vaccine was given, the manufacturer's name and lot number, where the vaccine was administered, and the professional title (MD, RN) of the person administering the vaccine. It also commands the federal government to improve existing vaccines and develop safer vaccines. The compensation portion of the law is an alternative to suing vaccine manufacturers and physicians when children or adults are damaged or die from reactions to mandated vaccines. It awards up to $250,000 if the individual dies, and other amounts for pain and suffering in the case of a living (but brain damaged) child.[854]

Although doctors are required by federal law to inform parents about vaccine risks, very few do. Yet vaccine manufacturers place warnings on vaccine containers indicating who *should not* receive vaccinations. They also publish a list of adverse reactions that may occur. This information is available by asking your doctor to show you these warning labels *before* the vaccines are given or by visiting your library and reviewing the *Physician's Desk Reference* (PDR).

Vaccine authorities do not officially recognize several conditions that may place your child at greater risk despite extensive anecdotal evidence and scientific literature published by vaccine researchers throughout the world. For example, additional caution may be warranted if the child is ill with anything, including a runny nose, cough, ear infection, diarrhea, or has recently recovered from an illness, or if the child was born prematurely or with low birth weight.[855] Vaccines may also be contraindicated for some people with special conditions not listed above. If you suspect that you or your child may be high risk for a vaccine reaction, *investigate!*

Reporting Vaccine Reactions: Many doctors refuse to report vaccine reactions despite the legal requirement to do so. According to Barbara Loe Fisher of the National Vaccine Information Center (NVIC), "the will and intent of Congress in enacting the National Vaccine Injury Act of 1986 is being subverted. This subversion is resulting in an appalling underreporting of vaccine reactions and deaths... [There is also] a lack of recordkeeping and/or willingness on the part of physicians to divulge the manufacturer's name and lot number when a reaction occurs."[856] An NVIC survey in seven states revealed that only 28 out of 159 doctors (18%) said they inform the government when a child suffers a serious health problem following vaccinations (Figure 30).[857] In New York, only one doctor out of 40 reported vaccine adverse events to the government.[858]

According to NVIC, doctors often justify their refusal to report vaccine reactions by merely claiming the shot had nothing to do with the child's injury or death. Some pediatricians may actually believe this, because they quote vaccine policymakers in the AAP and CDC who tell them that the vaccine is completely safe.[859] However, the fear of being sued for failing to warn parents of the potential dangers and contraindications may also be a consideration.

The following excerpts from parents and relatives of vaccine-damaged children illustrate how doctors can easily dismiss apparent vaccine reactions and thus justify not reporting them:

"We lost our beautiful, precious and adored four-month-old son 26 hours after receiving the DPT vaccination and oral polio [vaccine] at his well-baby check-up... Our son's behavior patterns changed after the shot... He was staring, looked spacey, only took short naps, vomited his bottle... The doctor was insistent that this was a SIDS death." *The doctor would not report this reaction. He did not feel that it was related to the vaccine.*

"My grandson had his 1st DPT shot and oral polio [vaccine] at his two month well-baby check-up. Within 21 hours he was dead. After the shot he started [high-pitched screaming]... My grandson began projectile vomiting and continued the high-pitched crying... At 7 a.m. my daughter awoke and found my grandson to have a purple color on one side of his face, clenched fists, blood coming from his nose and mouth, and not breathing. My grandson was dead. I have promised my daughter that his death will not be in vain and just another statistic labeled SIDS." *The doctor would not report this reaction. He did not feel that it was related to the vaccine.*[860]

Note: If the doctor refuses to report a vaccine reaction, parents may file their own report by calling: **1-800-822-7967.**

Figure 30:

Do Doctors Report Vaccine Reactions?

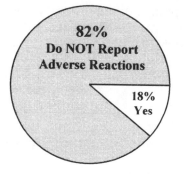

Copyright © 2002, NZM

A survey in seven states revealed that only 28 out of 159 doctors (18%) said they make a report to the government when a child suffers a serious health problem following vaccination. Source: National Vaccine Information Center.

What Causes a Vaccine Reaction? When children receive their shots from a "hot lot" (an improperly prepared and dangerous batch of vaccine that bypassed the safety testing system) they are especially susceptible to the inherent risks of the vaccine. Several studies indicate that children do not have to receive a shot from a "hot lot" in order to be at risk. Instead, certain children appear to be "anatomically susceptible," or genetically predisposed to having a reaction to the vaccine.[861,862] Also, many parents are unaware that potentially dangerous reactions even exist, so they fail to remain alert for neurological signs and other symptoms in their babies following their shots. However, *Pediatrics* published a study in which parents were specifically asked to observe any change in their baby's behavior or physical condition after a shot; only seven percent were able to report no reactions at all.[863]

Where Do Coroners Stand? Doctors and pediatricians are not the only instruments of the Medical-Industrial Complex who are likely to deny the existence of vaccine reactions and cover up the truth. Medically trained coroners are also members of this group. Many are highly skilled in the art of subterfuge. Rarely is the vaccination ever listed as the cause of death. Instead, they use impressive terms to falsify the death certificate: cardiac arrest, possible myocarditis; bronchial bilateral pneumonia;[864] septicemia due to septic tonsillitis; lymphatic leukemia; streptococcal cellulitis; tubercular meningitis; infantile paralysis; and SIDS, to name a few.[865]

When one mother, whose son died four days after his 2nd polio shot, studied his provisional autopsy report, she noted that there were major findings of myocarditis and hepatitis, and that the polio virus had been isolated in his diseased organs—conditions not inconsistent with a vaccine reaction. But when she questioned the pathology department's initial conclusion—sudden infant death syndrome—and requested additional tests to determine whether the polio virus was a wild or vaccine strain, she was led into a nine year battle with the CDC to secure the results. Medical authorities were eventually forced to concede the truth. The official death certificate listed the cause of death as "myocarditis, due to type 2 polio virus, due to oral Sabin polio vaccine."[866]

Promoting Vaccine Safety: The National Vaccine Advisory Committee (NVAC) was created by the Department of Health and Human Services (HHS), after Congress ordered HHS "to develop and disseminate vaccine information materials for distribution by health care providers." This material was to include information on adverse reactions, contraindications, and the availability of a federal no-fault compensation program for those who are injured or die from a mandated vaccine. Congress believed then, as it does now, that parents are entitled to such information before their children receive vaccinations. Still, this legal requisite was ignored for several years by vaccine authorities until the NVIC threatened to sue HHS on behalf of parents of vaccination-aged children.[867]

Because HHS failed to publish the required information, high risk children who **should not** have received one or more of the vaccines may have suffered from avoidable brain damage, permanent disabilities, and death. And parents whose children were injured or died from one or more of the vaccines during this period may have been unaware of their right to seek compensation. Vaccine guidelines were eventually submitted by the advisory committee (after the Congressional deadline) but were rejected by NVIC on the grounds that they "failed to meet even minimal standards of scientific rigor, candor, and fairness." Vaccine risks were systematically understated or ignored. For example, the proposed guidelines stated that "a few people will have a serious problem," but they did not mention that a "serious problem" could mean permanent brain damage or death. The guidelines also revealed a selective use of scientific data, downplayed the true rates of adverse reactions, and gave inconsistent, incomplete, inaccurate, and potentially dangerous information regarding contraindications.[868]

According to Barbara Loe Fisher, who chaired the subcommittee on adverse reactions for the NVAC, "even though Congress gave the NVAC a dual mission: 'to achieve optimal prevention of human infectious disease through immunization' and 'to achieve optimal prevention against adverse reactions to vaccines,' I had observed that the majority of NVAC time was spent discussing how to promote vaccination. The equally important goal of identifying ways to prevent vaccine reactions appears to be a subject that causes discomfort among many committee members, is viewed as an obstacle to promoting vaccination, and is generally given little time or in-depth treatment."[869] Fisher also noted that "not only is there a lack of concern about the subject of vaccine reactions on the part of some committee members, but there is a deliberate attempt to deny the reality of vaccine reactions, deaths and injuries... [Committee members need] to spend more time trying to find ways to solve problems associated with preventing vaccine reactions rather than trying to find ways to reword subcommittee reports to deny the existence of [children who were damaged or killed by a vaccine]."[870]

Furthermore, two prominent doctors believed to be impartial advisors to HHS were charged with failing to disclose conflicts of interest after it was discovered that they (and the research programs that support them) were paid by vaccine manufacturers over $800,000 in expert witness and consulting fees and research grants.[871] More recently, on June 15, 2000, Congress held a hearing on *Conflicts of Interest and Vaccine Development.* In this hearing, it was revealed that two advisory committees associated with the FDA and CDC "make vaccine policies that affect every child in this country."[872] Yet, members of these committees own stock in drug companies that make vaccines. One member, who sat on the CDC's vaccine advisory committee, was paid by the pharmaceutical industry "to travel around the country and teach doctors that vaccines are safe."[873] He recommended adding the rotavirus vaccine to the national immunization schedule despite holding a patent on a rotavirus vaccine![874] This vaccine was hurried onto the market then quietly removed when it was found to be extremely dangerous.[875]

Congressional chairman Dan Burton wrote to HHS Secretary Donna Shalala requesting that HHS "implement policies to prevent members with conflicts of interest from sitting on the FDA and the CDC advisory committees."[876,877] A Congressional spokesperson told reporters "there are conflict of interest laws that are not being followed. If you're going to make a decision that affects public health, it should be well known that you own stock in the manufacturer of the product."[878] But the FDA and HHS made it clear that they had no intention of revising their financial disclosure policies.[879]

Claims for Compensation: The general public is essentially unaware of the true number of people (mostly children) who have been permanently damaged or killed by one or more of the vaccines. *Every year about 12,000 reports of adverse reactions to vaccines are made to the FDA.*[880] These figures include emergency hospitalizations, irreversible injuries, and deaths. Still, these numbers may be grossly underreported because the FDA estimates that 90 percent of doctors do not report reactions.[881,882] A confidential study conducted by Connaught Laboratories, a vaccine manufacturer, indicated that "a *fifty-fold* underreporting of adverse events" is likely.[883] Yet, even this figure may be conservative. According to Dr. David Kessler, former director of the FDA, "Only about one percent of serious events [adverse drug reactions] are reported."[884]

The general public is also essentially unaware of the amount of money awarded in these cases. In the last few years, *more than $1 BILLION* had already been granted for thousands of injuries and deaths caused by mandated vaccines.[885] Numerous cases are still pending. Awards were issued for permanent injuries that included learning disabilities, seizure disorders, mental retardation, paralysis, and numerous deaths, including many that were initially misclassified as sudden infant death syndrome (SIDS).

Who Pays for Compensation? In order to pay for vaccine injuries or deaths, Congress established a special tax on the sale of mandated vaccines. The fee on each vaccine corresponds to the anticipated funds needed to pay for injuries and deaths resulting from that vaccine. This fee is passed on to consumers. In other words, when moms and dads pay the doctor for vaccines, some of the money goes into this special fund to cover the possibility that their child may suffer a severe or fatal vaccine reaction.[886]

Are Vaccines Mandatory? Scare tactics, skewed statistics, and outright lies are often used by medical personnel and school officials to intimidate wavering parents into vaccinating their children. (Several examples of these *vaccine ploys* are documented on the following website: www.thinktwice.com/ploys.htm) In addition, many colleges now require new students to be fully vaccinated as a prerequisite to admission. The government may even deny welfare and other benefits to families who refuse vaccinations.[887,888] Many doctors and school authorities tell parents that state laws and school regulations require their children to receive mandated vaccines. However, *all states provide exemptions allowing parents to oppose mandated vaccines.* For further information on vaccine regulations, visit your state law library. You may also acquire a copy of your exact state law and a sample exemption letter by visiting the following website: www.thinktwice.com/laws.htm This extensive resource contains valuable information regarding vaccines.

Despite signing these waivers, some parents have been charged with child abuse for not vaccinating their children and were hustled into court with the threat of losing custody of their loved ones. Court officials, social workers, and even foster parents have tried to force injections on the children.[889,890] Ironically, some parents who did vaccinate their children have lost custody of them, and were accused of child abuse—"shaking baby syndrome"—when their babies had seizures, went into a coma, or died, following their shots.[891-894]

Authorities also argue that parents should vaccinate their children to protect society as a whole from epidemics. But if the vaccines offered true immunity only the unvaccinated would become ill. Therefore, decisions that affect your child's health should not be forced upon you by so-called experts who are neither willing nor able to take responsibility for their actions.

The Germ Theory: Some researchers believe that germs do not cause disease. If this is true, then the very roots of vaccine theory are flawed.[895] According to Dr. Antoine Bechamp, renowned scientist and bacteriologist, germs are an integral part of living cells. They remain dormant until the cell has completed its life cycle and begins to decay. Germs help to decompose the dying cell so that it may be eliminated from the body.[896,897] Dr. Robert Koch, another opponent of the germ theory, confirms Bechamp's explanation. He believes that if germs cause disease, then specific germs must a) be found in every case of the disease, and b) never be found apart from the disease. But germs do not conform to these requirements.[898]

According to the German bacteriologist, Guenther Enderlein, whose treatment techniques have been used in Europe for more than 50 years, certain bacteria take on multiple forms during a single life cycle (pleomorphism). Some microbial forms that live in the human body are, under certain conditions, associated with many of the worst chronic diseases known to humankind. But when a person is healthy, these microbes are helpful to the body's immune system and live with the other cells in a symbiotic relationship. However, any severe change or deterioration of the body's internal environment—the "terrain"—due to poor nutrition or other factors, could cause the microbes to change into disease-causing forms as they pass through different stages of their life cycle. Simply put, "the germ is nothing, the terrain is everything."[899]

Louis Pasteur, the French chemist and bacteriologist who had the greatest influence on the course of medicine and the medical concept of disease, initially believed that all disease was caused by external microbes that invaded the body. He claimed that healthy tissues were germ-free. However, before Pasteur died, he retreated from this view and admitted that the internal environment was the key, but his earlier ideas endured.[900] Even Rudolph Virchow, German pathologist and founder of cellular medicine, stated: "If I could live my life over again, I would devote it to proving that germs seek their natural habitat—'diseased' tissue—rather than being the cause of the 'diseased' tissue." And Dr. George White observed that "if the germ theory were founded on facts, there would be no living being to read what's written."[901]

Natural Immunity: These researchers and many others believe that a proper diet is essential to health. This means eating foods that are unrefined, organically grown, and preservative-free.[902-904] An improper diet overwhelms the system and leads to sickness, for disease is the cleansing effort of the body to rid itself of an excess of toxins and waste material.[905] Adequate rest and sanitary living conditions are also integral to health. According to Dr. Harold Buttram, when these requirements are met, "many diseases will pass as subclinical infections without acute illness, or if there is illness, it will be relatively mild."[906] Thus, natural immunity is best achieved by proper hygiene and wholesome living. Research also indicates that breastfed newborns have healthier immune systems than babies that are bottle-fed.[907-909] Other studies show that excessive sugar consumption may increase the incidence of infections and reduce the body's ability to defend against disease.[910,911]

Finally, parents who are disenchanted with the allopathic or medical approach to illness may wish to consult with naturopathic, chiropractic, and homeopathic doctors. These highly qualified and licensed health practitioners may be found in your telephone book.

Summary & Conclusion

A brief review of the data presented in this book indicates that:

1) Many of the vaccines were *not* the true cause of a decline in the incidence of the disease. Increased nutritional and sanitary measures probably deserve much of the credit. Several diseases may also have their own evolutionary cycles; the virulent nature of the virgin disease is transformed into a tame illness as members of the population are exposed to it and gain "herd" immunity.

2) *None* of the vaccines is able to confer genuine immunity. Often, the opposite is true; the vaccine *increases* the chance of contracting the disease. Vaccine "efficacy rates" can be misleading. They are often evaluated by measuring antibody levels—not by comparing infection rates in vaccinated and unvaccinated persons.[912]

3) All of the vaccines can produce side effects. Reactions range from soreness at the injection site to brain damage and death.

4) The long-term effects of *all* vaccines are unknown. Particularly distressing are the implications that vaccines can be devastating to the young child's immature immune system. Studies were presented showing impaired health protection following injections. Lowered physical defenses may be responsible for a new breed of autoimmune diseases. Other studies showed damage to the brain and nervous system following shots—post-vaccinal encephalitis. This, in turn, causes large numbers of children to grow up with physical, mental and emotional disabilities of varying degrees. All of these conditions affect the individual, his or her family, and society as well.

5) Several of the vaccines can be especially dangerous. Nevertheless, the Medical-Industrial Complex continues to maintain its deceptive practice of disregarding vaccine reactions. In fact, medical officials have suggested that they are justified in administering new and unproven vaccines by claiming it is unethical to withhold them!?[913] Meanwhile, creative propaganda on the merits of vaccinations remains a lucrative ploy. For example, the AMA admits that "adult vaccines need a gimmick." CDC physicians have suggested a catchy slogan, like "Vaccines are not just kid stuff."[914] Hollywood stars, such as Bill Cosby and Whoopi Goldberg, have been recruited

as well. They have been seen and heard on TV and radio warning parents to "Vaccinate, before it's too late."[915] In England, the National Health Service pays a "bonus" to doctors with documented vaccination rates above specified percentages.[916] Of course, in the United States informal pressures and inducements to obey authority are not enough. Our medical policymakers have lobbied for laws against freedom of choice. Their patterns of coercion and denial are notorious among the enlightened members of the population, including parents who question vaccines, though sadly their awakenings may have cost them dearly—often the health or life of their own child.

Vaccinations are not the only basis for the unfortunate conditions noted throughout the text. Personal maladies and social ills have several causes. Nor are all members of the medical establishment callous and uncaring. Many are simply unaware of the true extent of damage being caused by vaccines. They sincerely believe that only good can come from being injected with foreign germs and toxic matter. But in a free country like the United States of America, no one should be compelled to submit to dangerous health practices against their will. Health and illness are personal experiences belonging to the people undergoing them. Nobody else has the right to dictate how they will be managed. That choice is the individual's alone, or belongs to the legitimate guardians of a dependent child.

Some mothers have long suspected that vaccines may not be appropriate for their children, but they worry about whether they can make the decision not to vaccinate and still be strong enough to face their pediatrician, family and friends. Many fathers are also uneasy when questioning society and the status quo. They don't want to be considered "soft" on the vaccine issue. But the decision regarding whether or not to vaccinate is the parent's alone. It must not be based upon irrational factors. Instead, this choice should be made only after examining credible evidence from several sources. In addition, critical thinking should be exercised when interpreting information. I encourage parents to substantiate all of the references in this book and to research this topic even further if questions still remain. As parents, you are entitled to—and responsible for obtaining —the facts about the benefits and risks of vaccinating your children.

Notes

1. Thomson, William A. R., *Black's Medical Dictionary* (Totawa, NJ: Barnes & Noble Books, 1987), p. 716.
2. *The World Book Encyclopedia,* Volume 11 (1994), p. 91.
3. Volk, W.A., et al. *Basic Microbiology, 4th edition.* (Philadelphia, PA: J.B. Lippincott Co., 1980), p. 455.
4. *Physician's Desk Reference* (PDR); 55th edition. (Montvale, NJ: Medical Economics, 2001), p. 778.
5. Burnet, M., et al. *The Natural History of Infectious Disease* (New York, NY: Cambridge University Press, 1972), p. 16.
6. See Note 4.
7. Neustaedter, R. *The Vaccine Guide.* (Berkeley, CA: North Atlantic Books, 1996), pp. 107-108.
8. See Note 4.
9. Baby Center. "The Polio Vaccine (0-12 months)." www.babycenter. com/refcap/155.html?CP_bid=
10. Moskowitz, Richard, MD. "Immunizations: The Other Side." *Mothering* (Spring 1984), p. 36.
11. Houchaus. "Ueber Poliomyelitis acuta." *Munch Med Wochenschr* 1909; 56:353-55.
12. Lambert, S.M. "A yaws campaign and an epidemic of poliomyelitis in Western Samoa." *J Trop Med Hyg* 1936; 39:41-46.
13. Lindsay, K.W., et al. *Neurology and Neurosurgery Illustrated.* (Edinburgh/London/New York: Churchill Livingstone, 1986), pp. 100, Figure 15.2. Polio incidence rates obtained from National Morbidity Reports.
14. McCloskey, B.P. "The relation of prophylactic inoculations to the onset of poliomyletis." *Lancet* (April 18, 1950), pp. 659-63.
15. Geffen, D.H. "The incidence of paralysis occurring in London children within four weeks after immunization." *Med Officer* 1950; 83:137-40.
16. Martin, J.K. "Local paralysis in children after injections." *Arch Dis Child* 1950; 25:1-14.
17. Sutter, Roland W., et al. "Attributable risk of DTP (Diphtheria and Tetanus Toxoids and Pertussis Vaccine) injection in provoking paralytic poliomyelitis during a large outbreak in Oman." *Journal of Infectious Diseases* 1992; 165:444-449.
18. Strebel, Peter M., et al. "Intramuscular injections within 30 days of immunization with oral poliovirus vaccine—a risk factor for vaccine-associated paralytic poliomyelitis." *New England J of Med* (February 23, 1995), pp. 500+.
19. Mendelsohn, Robert. *How to Raise a Healthy Child...In Spite of Your Doctor.* (Ballantine Books, 1984), pp. 231 and 251.
20. Alderson, Michael. *International Mortality Statistics* (Washington, DC: Facts on File, 1981), pp. 177-78.
21. Ibid.
22. See Note 19.
23. McBean, Eleanor. *The Poisoned Needle.* (Mokelumne Hill, California: Health Research, 1974), p. 140. Data taken from government statistics, as reported in an Associated Press dispatch from Boston (August 30, 1955).
24. Allen, Hannah. *Don't Get Stuck: The Case Against Vaccinations.* (Oldsmar, Florida: Natural Hygiene Press, 1975), p. 146.
25. See Note 23, p. 142.
26. Ibid.
27. Ibid., p. 140.
28. Ibid.
29. See Note 23, p. 144. As reported by Saul Pett in an Associated Press dispatch from Pittsburgh (October 11, 1954).
30. See Note 23, pp. 142-45.
31. Hearings Before the Committee on Interstate and Foreign Commerce, House of Representatives, 87th Congress, 2nd Session on HR 10541. May 1962, pp. 94-112.
32. Los Angeles County Health Index: Morbidity and Morality, Reportable Diseases.
33. Bayly, M. Beddow, *The Case Against Vaccination* (York Road, London: William H. Taylor & Sons, Ltd., Printers, June 1936), p. 4.
34. *Washington Post* (September 24, 1976).
35. American Academy of Pediatrics, *Report of the Committee on Infectious diseases: 1986* (Elk Grove Village, Illinois: AAP), pp. 284-85.
36. Strebel, Peter M., et al. "Epidemiology of poliomyletis in U.S. one decade after the last reported case of indigenous wild virus associated disease," *Clinical Infectious Diseases* (CDC, February 1992), pp. 568-79.
37. Ibid.

38. Institute of Medicine. "An evaluation of poliomyelitis vaccine policy options." *IOM Publication 88-04* (Washington DC: National Academy of Sciences, 1988).

39. Vaccine Adverse Event Reporting System (VAERS), Rockville, MD.

40. IOS. "The Polio vaccine coverup—OPV Vaccine Report: Document #14." www.ios.com/~w1066/poliov6.html

41. See Note 36, p. 568.

42. Gorman, Christine. "When the vaccine causes polio." *Time* (October 30, 1995), p. 83.

43. Shaw, Donna. "Unintended casualties in war on polio." *Philadelphia Inquirer* (June 6, 1993), p. A1.

44. U.S. Department of Health and Human Services. "Polio: What You Need to Know." (Atlanta, GA: CDC, October 15, 1991), p. 3.

45. See Note 4, p. 780.

46. Ibid.

47. O'Hern, E.M. *Profiles: Pioneer Women Scientists.* (Bethesda, MD: National Institutes of Health.)

48. Curtis, Tom, et al. "Scientist's Polio Fear Unheeded: How U.S. Researcher's Warning Was Silenced." *The Houston Post* 1992, pp. A1 and A12.

49. Sweet, B.H. and Hilleman M.R. "The Vacuolating Virus: SV-40." As cited in "The polio vaccine and simian virus 40" by Moriarty, T.J. www.chronicillnet.org/online/bensweet.html

50. See Note 48.

51. Shah, K and Nathanson, N. "Human exposure to SV40." *American Journal of Epidemiology*, 1976; 103:1-12.

52. Curtis, Tom. "The origin of AIDS: A startling new theory attempts to answer the question 'Was it an act of God or an act of man.'" *Rolling Stone* (March 19, 1992), p. 57.

53. Bookchin, D., and Schumaker, J. "Tainted Polio Vaccine Still Carries Its Threat 40 Years Later." *The Boston Globe* (January 26, 1997).

54. See Notes 51 and 52.

55. Innis, M.D. "Oncogenesis and poliomyelitis vaccine." *Nature*, 1968; 219:972-73.

56. Soriano, F., et al. "Simian virus 40 in a human cancer." *Nature*, 1974; 249:421-24.

57. Weiss, A.F., et al. "Simian virus 40-related antigens in three human meningiomas with defined chromosome loss." *Proceedings of the National Academy of Science* 1975; 72(2):609-13.

58. Scherneck, S., et al. "Isolation of a SV-40-like papovavirus from a human glioblastoma." *International Journal of Cancer* 1979; 24:523-31.

59. Stoian, M., et al. "Possible relation between viruses and oromaxillofacial tumors. II. Research on the presence of SV40 antigen and specific antibodies in patients with oromaxillofacial tumors." *Virologie*, 1987; 38:35-40.

60. Stoian, M., et al. "Possible relation between viruses and oromaxillofacial tumors. II. Detection of SV40 antigen and of anti-SV40 antibodies in patients with parotid gland tumors." *Virologie*, 1987; 38:41-46.

61. Bravo, M.P., et al. "Association between the occurrence of antibodies to simian vacuolating virus 40 and bladder cancer in male smokers." *Neoplasma*, 1988; 35:285-88.

62. O'Connell, K., et al. "Endothelial cells transformed by SV40 T-antigen cause Kaposi's sarcoma-like tumors in nude mice." *American Journal of Pathology*, 1991; 139(4):743-49.

63. Weiner, L.P., et al. "Isolation of virus related to SV40 from patients with progressive multifocal leukoencephalopathy." *New England Journal of Medicine*, 1972; 286:385-90.

64. Tabuchi, K. "Screening of human brain tumors for SV-40-related T-antigen." *International Journal of Cancer* 1978; 21:12-17.

65. Meinke, W., et al. "Simian virus 40-related DNA sequences in a human brain tumor." *Neurology* 1979; 29:1590-94.

66. Krieg, P., et al. "Episomal simian virus 40 genomes in human brain tumors." *Proceedings of the National Academy of Sciences* 1981; 78(10):6446-50.

67. Krieg, P., et al. "Cloning of SV40 genomes from human brain tumors." *Virology* 1984; 138:336-40.

68. Geissler, E. "SV40 in human intracranial tumors: passenger virus or oncogenic 'hit-and-run' agent?" *Z Klin Med*, 1986; 41:493-95.

69. Geissler, E. "SV40 and Human Brain Tumors." *Progress in Medical Virology*, 1990; 37:211-222.

70. Bergsagel, D.J., et al. "DNA sequences similar to those of simian virus 40 in ependymomas and choroid plexus tumors of childhood." *New England Journal of Medicine*, 1992; 326:988-93.

71. Martini, M., et al. "Human Brain Tumors and Simian Virus 40." *Journal of the National Cancer Institute*, 1995; 87(17):1331.

72. Lednicky, J.A., et al. "Natural Simian Virus 40 Strains are Present in Human Choroid Plexus and Ependymoma Tumors." *Virology*, 1995; 212(2):710-17.

73. Tognon, M., et al. "Large T Antigen Coding Sequence of Two DNA Tumor Viruses, BK and SV-40, and Nonrandom Chromosome Changes in Two Gioblastoma Cell Lines." *Cancer Genetics and Cytogenics*, 1996; 90(1): 17-23.

74. *Journal of the National Cancer Institute*, 1999; 91(2):169-175.

75. See Notes 63-74.

76. Carbone, M., et al. "SV-40 Like Sequences in Human Bone Tumors." *Oncogene*, 1996, 13(3):527-35.

77. Pass, H.I., Carbone, M., et al. "Evidence For and Implications of SV-40 Like Sequences in Human Mesotheliomas." *Important Advances in Oncology*, 1996, pp. 89-108.

78. Rock, Andrea. "The Lethal Dangers of the Billion Dollar Vaccine Business." *Money* (December 1996), p. 161.

79. Ibid.

80. Carlsen, William. "Rogue virus in the vaccine: Early polio vaccine harbored virus now feared to cause cancer in humans." *San Francisco Chronicle* (July 15, 2001), p. 7. Research by Susan Fisher,

epidemiologist, Loyola University Medical Center.

81. Rosa, F. W., et al. "Absence of antibody response to simian virus 40 after inoculation with killed-poliovirus vaccine of mothers offspring with neurological tumors." *New England Journal of Medicine,* 1988; 318:1469.

82. Rosa, F. W., et al. Response to: "Neurological tumors in offspring after inoculation of mothers with killed poliovirus vaccine." *New England Journal of Medicine,* 1988; 319:1226.

83. See Note 52, p. 58.

84. Martini, F., et al. "SV-40 Early Region and Large T Antigen in Human Brain Tumors, Peripheral Blood Cells, and Sperm Fluids from Healthy Individuals." *Cancer Research,* 1996, 56(20):4820-4825.

85. See Note 78, p. 163.

86. Ibid.

87. See Note 84.

88. Fisher, Barbara. "Vaccine safety consumer group cites conflict of interest in government report on cancer and contaminated polio vaccine link." *National Vaccine Information Center (NVIC);* Press Release (January 27, 1998).

89. See Note 80, p. 10.

90. Ibid., pp. 10 and 13.

91. See Note 43, pp. 57-58.

92. Koprowksi, H. "Tin anniversary of the development of live virus vaccine." *Journal of the American Medical Association* 1960; 174:972-76.

93. Hayflick, L., Koprowski, H., et al. "Preparation of poliovirus vaccines in a human fetal diploid cell strain." *American J Hyg* 1962; 75: 240-258.

94. Koprowski, Hilary. In a letter sent to the Congressional Health and Safety Subcommittee, April 14, 1961.

95. Ibid.

96. See Note 78, p. 159.

97. Ibid.

98. Ibid.

99. Curtis, Tom. "Expert says test vaccine: backs check of polio stocks for AIDS virus." *The Houston Post* (March 22, 1992), p. A-21.

100. See Note 80, p. 5.

101. Essex, M., et al. "The origin of the AIDS virus." *Scientific American,* 1988; 259:64-71.

102. Karpas, A. "Origin and Spread of AIDS." *Nature,* 1990; 348:578.

103. Kyle, W. S. "Simian retroviruses, poliovaccine, and origin of AIDS." *Lancet,* 1992; 339:600-601.

104. Elswood, B.F. and Stricker, R.B. "Polio vaccines and the origin of AIDS." *Medical Hypothesis,* vol. 42, 1994, pp. 347-354.

105. Myers, G., et al. "The emergence of simian/human immunodeficiency viruses." *AIDS Res Human Retro* 1992: 8:373-86.

106. Workshop on Simian Virus-40 (SV-40): A Possible Human Polyomavirus. (National Vaccine Information Center, January 27-28, 1997.) www.909shot.com/polio197.htm (Includes a summary of evidence presented at the Eighth Annual Houston Conference on AIDS.)

107. Martin, Brian. "Polio vaccines and the origin of AIDS: The career of a threatening idea." *Townsend Letter for Doctors* (January 1994), pp. 97-100.

108. Curtis, Tom. "Did a polio vaccine experiment unleash AIDS in Africa?" The Washington Post (April 5, 1992), pp. C3+.

109. See Note 52, pp. 54+.

110. See Notes 99 and 101-104.

111. See Note 52, pp. 106+.

112. See Note 4.

113. See Note 78, p. 163.

114. Reuters Health. "Polio outbreak in Hispaniola blamed on vaccine-derived poliovirus." *Reuters Medical News* (March 15, 2002). www.medscape.com/viewarticle/430159

115. "Problems with eradicating polio." *Science News* (November 25, 2000), p. 348.

116. Yoshida, H., et al. *Lancet* (October 28, 2000).

117. Crainic, R., et al. "Polio virus with natural recombinant genomes isolated from vaccine associated paralytic poliomyelitis." *Virology* 1993; 196:199-208.

118. See Note 2, Volume 19, p. 182.

119. Frick, L. "Tetanus." *Gale Encyclopedia of Alternative Medicine* (2001). www.findarticles.com/cf_dls/g2603/0007/2603000702/print.jhtml

120. Skudder, P.A., et al. "Current status of tetanus control: importance of human tetanus-immune globulin." *Journal of the American Medical Association* 1964; 188:625-627.

121. See Note 4, pp. 878-879.

122. McComb, J.A., et al. "Passive-active immunization with tetanus immune globulin (human)." *New England Journal of Medicine* 1963; 268:857-862.

123. Mortimer, E. "Immunization against infectious disease." *Science,* Volume 200 (May 26, 1978), p. 905.

124. See Note 10, p. 36.

125. See Note 7, p. 100.

126. Dunavan, C.P. "Blindsided by tetanus." *Discover/The Gale Group and LookSmart,* January 2000. www.findarticles.com/cf_dls/m1511/1_21/58398797/ print.jhtml

127. CDC. "Summary of notifiable diseases, United States, 1999." *MMWR* 1999 (Published April 6, 2001); 48 (No. 53):84-90.

128. Mackay, I. "Tetanus." *Virology Down Under,* 2001. www.uq.edu.au/vdu/tetanus.htm

129. National Advisory Committee on Immunization. *Canadian Immunization Guide* (Ottawa: Canada Communication Group Publishing, 1993), p. 116.

130. CDC. "Tetanus: United States, 1985-1986. *MMWR* 1987; 36:477-481.
131. CDC. "Tetanus: United States, 1987-1988. *MMWR* 1990; 39:37-41.
132. Oxygen Media. "Drugs: tetanus antitoxin (systemic)." *ThriveOnline,* 2001. www.thriveonline. oxygen.com/medical/library/drugs/203079b.html
133. See Note 128.
134. CDC. Figures extracted from several *Morbidity and Mortality Weekly Reports.*
135. See Note 127, p. xv.
136. Blumstein, G.I., et al. "Peripheral neuropathy following tetanus toxoid administration." *Journal of the American Medical Association* 1966; 198:1030-1031.
137. Wilson, G.S. "Allergic manifestations: post-vaccinal neuritis." *The Hazards of Immunization* (1967), pp. 153-156.
138. Tsairis, P., et al. "Natural history of brachial plexus neuropathy." *Archives of Neurology* 1972; 27:109-117.
139. Schlenska, G.K. "Unusual neurological complications following tetanus toxoid administration." *Journal of Neurology* 1977; 215:299-302.
140. Pollard, J.D., et al. "Relapsing neuropathy due to tetanus toxoid." *Journal of Neurological Science* 1978; 37:113-125.
141. Quast, U., et al. "Mono- and polyneuritis after tetanus vaccination." *Devel Bio Stand* 1979; 43:25-32.
142. Eibl, M., et al. "Abnormal T-lymphocyte subpopulations in healthy subjects after tetanus booster immunizations," *New England Journal of Medicine* (November 26, 1981):1307-1313.
143. Buttram, H.E. and Hoffman, J.C. "Bringing Vaccines Into Perspective." *Mothering* (Winter 1985), p. 30.
144. Reinstein, L., et al. "Peripheral neuropathy after multiple tetanus toxoid injections." *Archives Phys Med Rehabilitation* 1982; 63:332-334.
145. Fenichel, G.M. "Neurological complications of tetanus toxoid." *Archives of Neurology* 1983; 40:390.
146. Holliday, P.L., et al. "Polyradiculoneuritis secondary to immunization with tetanus and diphtheria toxoids." *Archives of Neurology* 1983; 40:390.
147. Rutledge, S.L., et al. "Neurologic complications of immunizations. *Journal of Pediatrics* 1986; 109:917-924.
148. CDC. "Adverse events following immunization." *MMWR* 1985; 34(3):43-47.
149. CDC. "Recommendations of the immunization practices advisory committee (ACIP): diphtheria, tetanus and pertussis: guidelines for vaccine prophylaxis and other preventive measures." *MMWR* 1985; 34:405-426.
150. CDC. "Update: vaccine side effects, adverse reactions, contraindications, and precautions." *MMWR* 1996; 45:22-31.
151. Kroger, G., et al. "Tetanusimpfung: Vertraglichkeit und Vermeidung von Nebenreaktionen." [Tetanus vaccination: tolerance and avoidance of adverse reactions.] *Klininische Wochenschrift* 1986; 64:767-775.
152. Newton, N., et al. "Guillain-Barré syndrome after vaccination with purified tetanus toxoid." *S Med J* 1987; 80: 1053-1054.
153. Schwartz, G., et al. "Acute midbrain syndrome as an adverse reaction to tetanus immunization." *Intensive Care Medicine* 1988; 15:53-54.
154. Jawad, A.S., et al. "Immunisation triggering rheumatoid arthritis?" *Annals of Rheumatic Disease* 1989; 48:174.
155. Read, S.J., et al. "Acute transverse myelitis after tetanus toxoid vaccination." *Lancet* 1992; 339:1111-1112.
156. Topaloglu, H., et al. "Optic neuritis and myelitis after booster tetanus toxoid vaccination." *Lancet* 1992; 339:178-179.
157. Institute of Medicine. *Adverse Events Associated with Childhood Vaccines: Evidence Bearing on Causality.* (Washington, DC: National Academy Press, 1994).
158. Regamey, R.H. Die Tetanus-Schutzimpfung. [Tetanus immunization in *Handbook of Immunization.*] In Herrlick, A., ed. *Handbuch Schutzimpfungen.* (Berlin: Springer, 1965).
159. Staak, M., et al. Zur problematik anaphylaktischer Reaktionen nach aktiver Tetanus-Immunisierung. [Anaphylactic reaction following active tetanus immunization.] *Deutsche Medizinische Wochenschrift* 1973; 98:110-111.
160. Kemp, T., et al. "Is infant immunization a risk factor for childhood asthma or allergy?" *Epidemiology* 1997; 8(6):678-680.
161. Hurwitz, E.L., et al. "Effects of diphtheria-tetanus-pertussis or tetanus vaccination on allergies and allergy-related respiratory symptoms among children and adolescents in the United States." *Journal of Manipulative and Physiological Therapeutics* 2000; 23:1-10.
162. See Note 142.
163. See Note 143.
164. See Note 157.
165. Ibid.
166. See Note 160.
167. See Note 161.
168. Fisher, B.L. *The Consumer's Guide to Childhood Vaccines.* (Vienna, VA: National Vaccine Information Center, 1997), p. 18.
169. See Note 10, p. 34.
170. See Note 2, Volume 13, p. 345.
171. Krishnamurthy, K.A., et al. "Measles a dangerous disease: a study of 1000 cases in Madurai." *Indian Pediatrics,* 1974: 267-71.
172. See Note 168, pp. 17-18.

173. Ibid.
174. Sommer, A., et al. "Increased risk of respiratory disease and diarrhea in children with pre-existing mild vitamin A deficiency." *American Journal of Clinical Nutrition* 1984; 40:1090-95.
175. Sommer, A., et al. "Impact of vitamin A supplementation on childhood mortality: a randomized clinical trial." *Lancet* 1986; 1:1169-73.
176. Barclay, A.J.G., et al. "Vitamin A supplements and mortality related to measles: a randomised clinical trial." *British Medical Journal* (January 31, 1987), pp. 294-96.
177. Keusch, G.T. "Vitamin A supplements—too good to be true." *New England Journal of Medicine* (October 4, 1990), p. 986.
178. Frieden, T.R., et al. "Vitamin A levels and severity of measles: New York City." *Am J Dis Child* 1992; 146:182-86.
179. *Pediatric Nursing* (September/October 1996).
180. U.S. Department of Health and Human Services. "Measles, Mumps, and Rubella: What You Need to Know." (Atlanta, GA: CDC, October 15, 1991), p. 1.
181. See Note 19, pp. 236-37.
182. See Note 7, p. 142.
183. See Note 181, p. 237.
184. Ibid.
185. See Note 20, pp. 182-183.
186. FDA. "FDA workshop to review warnings, use instructions, and precautionary information [on vaccines]." (Rockland, Maryland: FDA, September 18, 1992), p. 27.
187. See Note 19, p. 238.
188. CDC. "Measles." *MMWR* 1989; 38:329-330.
189. Resnick, S.K. "Should you vaccinated against measles?" *Natural Health* (January/February 1992), p. 30.
190. Gold, E. "Current progress in measles eradication in the United States." *Infect Med* 1997; 14(4):297-300, 310.
191. CDC. "U.S. Childhood Immunization Update: Measles." (March 1997).
192. CDC. "Measles—United States, 1999." *MMWR* 2000; 49(25): 557-560.
193. See Note 4, p. 1884.
194. Thompson, N.P. Wakefield, A.J. et al. "Is measles vaccination a risk factor for inflammatory bowel disease?" *Lancet* 1995; 345:1071-1074.
195. CDC. Cited in Haney, D.Q. "Wave of infant measles stems from '60s vaccinations." *Albuquerque Journal* (November 23, 1992), p. B3.
196. CDC. "Babies of vaccinated moms more susceptible to measles." *Pediatrics* (November 1999).
197. Rizetto, M., et al. *Journal of Infectious Diseases* (January 1982), pp. 18-22.
198. National Coalition for Adult Immunization. "Facts about measles for adults." (November 8, 2000). www.nfid.org/factsheets/measlesadult.html
199. *Vaccine Injury Compensation.* Hearing Before the Subcommittee on Health and the Environment; 98th Congress, 2nd Session, (December 19, 1984), p. 110.
200. See Note 2, Volume 13, pp. 925-926.
201. See Note 19, pp. 234-236.
202. Ibid.
203. Ibid.
204. See Note 168, pp. 18-19.
205. U.S. Department of Health and Human Services. "Measles, Mumps, and Rubella: What You Need to Know." (Atlanta, GA: CDC, October 15, 1991), p. 1.
206. McKinley Health Center. "Mumps vaccine." *University of Illinois* (October 5, 1998). www.mckinley.uiuc.edu/health-info/dis-cond/vacimmun/ mumpsvac.html
207. CDC Fact Sheet. "Facts about mumps for adults." *National Coalition for Adult Immunization* (April 2000). www.nfid.org/factsheets/mumpsadult.html
208. See Notes 200, 201, 204, 205, and 206.
209. Diodati, Catherine. *Immunization: History, Ethrics, Law and Health.* (Windsor, Ontario, Canada: Integral Aspects Inc., 1999), p. 113.
210. Scheibner, Viera. *Vaccination: 100 Years of Orthodox Research Shows that Vaccines Represent a Medical Assault on the Immune System.* (Blackheath, NSW, Australia: Scheibner Publications, 1993), p. 98.
211. See Notes 209 and 210.
212. See Note 168, p. 19.
213. CDC. "Summary of notifiable diseases, United States, 1993." *MMWR* 1994; 42: No. 53.
214. See Note 4, p. 1976.
215. Minnesota Department of Health. Figures cited by Christina Abel, of the *Minnesota Vaccine Support Group,* in a February 10, 2001 email.
216. Kaplan, K.M., et al. "Further evidence of the changing epidemiology of a childhood vaccine-preventable disease." *Journal of the American Medical Association* 1988; 260(10):1434-1438.
217. See Note 210, p. 106.
218. Briss, P.A., et al. "Sustained transmission of mumps in a highly vaccinated population: assessment of vaccine failure and waning vaccine-induced immunity." *J of Infectious Diseases* 1994; 169:77-82.
219. See Note 4, p. 1976 and 168, pp. 18-19.
220. See Note 19, pp. 234-236; Note 168; Note 206.
221. CDC. "Mumps—United States, 1985-1988." *MMWR* 1989; 38:101-05.
222. Ibid.
223. See Note 4, pp. 1954 and 1977.
224. Helmke, K., et al. "Islet cell antibodies and the development of diabetes mellitus in relation to mumps infection and mumps vaccination." *Diabetologia* 1986; 29:30-33.

225. Fescharek, R., et al. "Measles-mumps vaccination in the FRG: an empirical analysis after 14 years of use. II. Tolerability and analysis of spontaneously reported side effects." *Vaccine* 1990; 8:446-456.

226. Pawlowski, B., et al. "Mumps vaccination and type-1 diabetes." *Deutsche Medizinische Wochenschrift* 1991; 116:635.

227. Adler, J.B., et al. "Pancreatitis caused by measles, mumps, and rubella vaccine." *Pancreas* 1991; 6:489-490.

228. Albonico, H., Klein, P., et al. "The immunization campaign against measles, mumps and rubella—coercion leading to a realm of uncertainty: medical objections to a continued MMR immunization campaign in Switzerland." *JAM* 1992; 9(1).

229. Maclaren, N., et al. "Is insulin-dependent diabetes mellitus environmentally induced?" *New England Journal of Medicine* 1992; 327:348-349.

230. See Note 39.

231. Miller, E., et al. "Risk of aseptic meningitis after measles, mumps, and rubella vaccine in U.K. children." *Lancet* 1993; 341:979.

232. Sawada, et al. *Lancet* 1993; 342:371.

233. See Note 157.

234. See Note 2, Volume 16, p. 506.

235. Ibid.

236. See Note 4, p. 1966.

237. Plotkin, S.A. "Development of RA 27/3 attenuated rubella virus grown in WI-38 cells." *Wistar Institute of Anatomy and Biology*. Cited in *International Symposium on Rubella Vaccines, London 1968; Symposium Series on Immunobiol. Standards* (Karger, Basel/New York, 1969); 11:249-260.

238. Hayflick, L., et al. "The serial cultivation of human diploid cell strains." *Exp. Cell Res.* 1961; 25:585-621.

239. Plotkin, S.A., et al. "Studies of immunization with living rubella virus. Trials in children with a strain cultured from an aborted foetus." *Amer. J. Dis. Child.* 1965; 110:381-389.

240. Hoskins, J.M., et al. "Behaviour of rubella virus in human diploid cell strains. I. Growth of virus. II. Studies of infected cells." *Arch. ges. Virusforsch* 1967; 21:283-296.

241. Hayflick, L. "The limited in vitro lifetime of human diploid cell strains." *Exp. Cell Res.* 1965; 37:614-636.

242. See Note 4, p. 1966.

243. Chantler, J.K., et al. "Persistent rubella infection and rubella-associated arthritis." *Lancet* (June 12, 1982):1323-1325.

244. Tingle, A.J., et al. "Prolonged arthritis, viraemia, hypogamma-globulinaemia, and failed seroconversion following rubella immunisation." *Lancet* 1984; 1:1475-1476.

245. Tingle, A.J., et al. "Postpartum rubella immunization: association with development of prolonged arthritis, neurological sequelae, and chronic rubella viremia." *Journal of Infectious Diseases* 1985; 152:606-612.

246. Tingle, A.J., et al. "Rubella-associated arthritis. Comparative study of joint manifestations associated with natural rubella infection and RA 27/3 rubella immunisation." *Annals of the Rheumatic Diseases* 1986; 45:110-114.

247. Kilroy, A.W., et al. "Two syndromes following rubella immunization." *Journal of the American Medical Association* 1970; 214:2287-2292.

248. Gilmarten, R.C., et al. "Rubella vaccine myeloradiculoneuritis." *Journal of Pediatrics* 1972; 80:406-412.

249. Schaffner, W., et al. "Polyneuropathy following rubella immunization: a follow-up study and review of the problem." *American Journal of Diseases of Children* 1974; 127:684-688.

250. Institute of Medicine. *Adverse Effects of Pertussis and Rubella Vaccines*. (Washington, DC: National Academy Press, 1991).

251. Mühlebach-Sponer, M., et al. "Intrathecal rubella antibodies in an adolescent with Guillain-Barré syndrome after mumps-measles-rubella vaccination." *European Journal of Pediatrics* 1994; 154:166.

252. See Note 39.

253. Coulter, Harris. "Childhood vaccinations and Juvenile-Onset (Type-1) diabetes." Congressional Testimony. *Committee on Appropriations, Subcommittee on Labor, Health and Human Services, Education, and Related Agencies.* (April 16, 1997).

254. Numazaki, K., et al. "Infection of cultured human fetal pancreatic islet cells by rubella virus." *American Journal of Clinical Pathology* 1989; 91:446-451.

255. Rayfield, E.J., et al. "Rubella virus-induced diabetes in the hamster." *Diabetes* (December 1986); 35:1278-1281.

256. Coyle, P.K., et al. "Rubella-specific immune complexes after congenital infection and vaccination." *Infection and Immunity* (May 1982); 36(2):498-503.

257. Lieberman, A.D. "The role of the rubella virus in the chronic fatigue syndrome." *Clinical Ecology* 1991; 7(3):51-54.

258. Allen, A.D. "Is RA27/3 rubella immunization a cause of Chronic Fatigue?" *Medical Hypotheses* 1988; 27:219.

259. Ibid., p. 220.

260. Ibid.

261. Ibid., p. 217.

262. These personal stories are typical of the unsolicited emails received by the *Thinktwice Global Vaccine Institute*. www.thinktwice.com

263. Cherry, J.D. "The 'new' epidemiology of measles and rubella." *Hospital Practice* (July 1980), pp. 56.

264. Spika, J.S., et al. "Rubella vaccination: a course becomes clear." *Canadian Medical Association Journal* (July 15, 1983); 129(2):106-110.

265. See Note 19, p. 240.
266. See Note 263, p. 55.
267. Bart, K.J., et al. "Universal immunization to interrupt rubella." *Review of Infectious Diseases* 1985; 7(1):S177-184.
268. Crowder, M., et al. "Rubella susceptibility in young women of rural East Texas: 1980 and 1985." *Texas Medicine* 1987; 83:43-47.
269. CDC. "Rubella and congenital rubella syndrome—United States, 1985-1988. *MMWR* 1989; 38:173-178.
270. CDC. "Current trends increase in rubella and congenital rubella syndrome—United States, 1988-1990." *MMWR Weekly* (February 15, 1991); 40(6):93-99.
271. Baker, B. "Rubella ready for possible worldwide eradication." *Pediatric News* 2000; 34(1):18.
272. CDC. "Summary of notifiable diseases, United States, 1995." *MMWR Weekly* (October 25, 1996); 44(53): 1-87.
273. CDC. "Notifiable diseases/deaths in selected cities weekly information." *MMWR Weekly* (January 5, 2001); 49(51): 1167-1174.
274. See Note 263, p. 55.
275. See Note 272.
276. Ibid.
277. "Rubella—Public Health Information Sheet." *March of Dimes Birth Defects Foundation* (White Plains, NY: October 1984). CDC data.
278. See Note 272.
279. Polk, B.F., et al. "An outbreak of rubella among hospital personnel." *New England Journal of Medicine* 1980; 303:541-545.
280. Orenstein, W.A., et al. "Rubella vaccine and susceptible hospital employees: poor physician participation." *Journal of the American Medical Association* (February 20, 1981); 245(7):711-713.
281. Sacks, J.J., et al. "Employee rubella screening program." *Journal of the American Medical Association* 1983; 249:2675-2678.
282. See Note 19, p. 241.
283. See Note 2, Volume 5 (1994), pp. 215-216.
284. Ibid.
285. Mackay, I. "Diphtheria: antitoxin." *Virology Down Under.* www.uq.edu. au/vdu/diphth.htm
286. Mortimer, E.A., et al. "Immunization against infectious disease." *Science* 1978; 200:902.
287. See Note 4, pp. 785-787.
288. Elben. *Vaccination Condemned,* (Los Angeles: Better Life Research, 1981), p. 57. Data taken from government statistics in New York.
289. *New York Health Bulletin* (February 1924).
290. Dublin, L., et al. *Twenty-Five Years of Health Progress* (New York: Metropolitan Life Insurance Company, 1937), p. 60.
291. See Note 4, p. 787.
292. CDC. Data published in several *Morbidity and Mortality Weekly Reports.*
293. CDC. "Summary of notifiable diseases, 1992." *MMWR* 1993; 41(55).
294. CDC. "Summary of notifiable diseases, 1999." *MMWR* (April 6, 2001); 48(53): 84-90.
295. CDC. "Notifiable diseases/deaths in selected cities weekly information." *MMWR Weekly* (January 5, 2001); 49(51):1167-1174.
296. See Note 20, pp. 161-162.
297. See Note 290, p. 56.
298. Bureau of Biologics. "Minutes of the 15th meeting of the panel of review of bacterial vaccines and toxoids with standards and potency." *Food and Drug Administration* (November 20-21, 1975).
299. See Note 4, p. 787, and Note 294.
300. Hardy, I.R., et al. "Current situation and control strategies for resurgence of diphtheria in newly independent states of the former Soviet Union." *Lancet* 1996; 347:1739-1744.
301. Prospero, E., et al. "Diphtheria: epidemiological update and review of prevention and control strategies." *European Journal of Epidemiology* 1997; 13:527-34.
302. Associated Press and Reuters. "FDA recalls diphtheria vaccine found to be too weak." *CNN Interactive* (January 29, 1999). www.cnn.com/health/9901/29/diphtheria.recall
303. Ibid.
304. See Note 10.
305. Ibid.
306. See Note 20, pp. 164-165.
307. Halperin, et al. "Persistence of Pertussis in an Immunized Population: Results of the Nova Scotia Enhanced Pertussis Surveillance Program," *Journal of Pediatrics* (Nov. 1989), pp. 686-693.
308. Pichichero, M.E., et al. "Diphtheria-Pertussis-Tetanus vaccine: reactogenicity of commercial products," *Pediatrics* (Feb. 1979), pp. 256-260.
309. U.S. Department of Health and Human Services. *20th Immunization Conference Proceedings, Dallas, Texas, May 6-9 1985* (October 1985), pp. 83-84.
310. *Vaccine Bulletin* (February 1987), p. 11.
311. Christie, D.C., et al. "The 1993 epidemic of pertussis in Cincinnati: resurgence of disease in a highly immunized population of children," *New England Journal of Medicine* (July 7, 1994), pp. 16-20.
312. FDA Press Release. "Newly formulated DTaP vaccine approved with only trace amounts of thimerosal." *FDA News* (March 7, 2001).
313. Murphy, Jamie. *What Every Parent Should Know About Childhood Immunization* (Boston, MA: Earth Healing Products, 1993), pp. 39-58.
314. Coulter, H.L. and Fisher, B.L. *A Shot in the Dark: Why the P in DPT Vaccination May be Hazardous to Your Child's Health,* (Garden City Park, NY: Avery Publishing Group, 1991), pp. 13-14.

315. Cherry, Brunell, et al, "Report of the task force on pertussis and pertussis immunization." *Pediatrics*, 81:6, pt. 2 (June 1988), p. 943.

316. Coulter, H.L. *Vaccination, Social Violence, and Criminality: The Medical Assault on the American Brain*, (Berkeley, CA: North Atlantic Books, 1990), p. xiv.

317. See Note 314, p. 11.

318. Ibid., pp. 32-34.

319. *Whooping Cough, the DPT Vaccine and Reducing Vaccine Reactions* (Vienna, VA., National Vaccine Information Center 1989), pp. 10-16.

320. *Immunization: Survey of Recent Research*, (United States Department of Health and Human Services, April 1983), p. 76.

321. "Nature and the Rates of Adverse Reactions Associated with DTP and DT Immunizations in Infants and Children," *Pediatrics*, Volume 68, No. 5 (November 1981).

322. Odent, M., et al. "Pertussis vaccination and asthma: is there a link?" *Journal of the American Medical Association* (August 24/31, 1994), pp. 592-593.

323. See Note 161.

324. Walker, A.M. "Does pertussis vaccine cause sudden infant death?" *Presentation for Institute of Medicine Workshop on Possible Adverse Consequences of Pertussis and Rubella Vaccines* (Washington, DC, May 14, 1990). Unpublished.

325. Fine and Chen. "Confounding in studies of adverse reactions to vaccines." *American Journal of Epidemiology*, 136, (1992), pp. 121-35.

326. See Note 314, p. 51.

327. Scheibnerova, V. *Cot Death as Due to Exposure to Non-Specific Stress and General Adaption Syndrome: Its Mechanisms and Prevention* (New South Wales, Australia: Association for Prevention of Cot Death, October 1990).

328. Scheibnerova, V. and Karlsson, L. *Association Between Non-specific Stress Syndrome, DPT Injections, and Cot Death* (Second Immunization Conference, Canberra, Australia, May 27-29, 1991).

329. See Note 210, pp. 59-70;225-235.

330. Torch, W.C. "Diphtheria-pertussis-tetanus (DPT) immunization: A potential cause of the sudden infant death syndrome (SIDS)," (American Academy of Neurology, 34th Annual Meeting, Apr 25 - May 1, 1982), *Neurology* 32(4), pt. 2.

331. *Vaccine Injury Compensation*. Hearing Before the Committee on Labor and Human Resources; 98th Congress, 2nd Session, (May 3, 1984), pp. 63-67.

332. See Note 314, pp. 208-210.

333. Cherry, J.D. "The future use of acellular pertussis vaccines in the U.S." *Vaccine Bulletin* (January 1987), p. 2.

334. Tompson, M. In *But Doctor, About That Shot...The Risks of Immunizations and How to Avoid Them*, by Mendelsohn, R.S. (Evanston, IL: The People's Doctor Newsletter, Inc., 1988), p. 96.

335. See Note 314, pp. 210-212.

336. Storsaeter, J., et al. "Mortality and morbidity from invasive bacterial infections during a clinical trial of acellular pertussis vaccines in Sweden." *Pediatric Infectious Disease Journal* 1988; 7: 637-645.

337. Blennow, M., et al. "Adverse reactions and serologic response to a booster dose of acellular pertussis vaccine in children immunized with acellular or whole-cell vaccine as infants." *Pediatrics* 1989; 84, pp. 62-67.

338. *AAP News Release* (April 15, 1992).

339. See Note 168, p. 37.

340. See Note 262.

341. Jacobson, I. M., Dienstag, J.L., et al. "Lack of effect of hepatitis B vaccine of T-cell phenotypes." *New England Journal of Medicine* 1984; 311(16):1030-1032.

342. See Note 157.

343. Alter, M.J., Hadler, S.C., et al. "The changing epidemiology of hepatitis B in the United States." *Journal of the American Medical Association* 1990; 263:1218-1222.

344. See Note 210, p. 3.

345. See Note 7, p. 171.

346. Stevens, C.E., et al. "Prospects for control of hepatitis B virus infection: implications of childhood vaccination and long-term protection." *Pediatrics* 1992; 90:170-173.

347. *New England Journal of Medicine*, July 24, 1986.

348. Street, A.C., et al. "Persistence of antibody in healthcare workers vaccinated against hepatitis B." *Infection Control and Hospital Epidemiology* 1990; 11:525-530.

349. Pasko, M.T., Beam, T.R. "Persistence of anti-HBs among health care personnel immunized with hepatitis B vaccine." *American Journal of Public Health* 1990; 80:590-593.

350. World Health Organization. "Hepatitis B vaccines: immunogenicity reappraised." *WHO Drug Information* 1994; 8(2).

351. Goffin, E., et al. "Acute hepatitis B infection after vaccination." *Lancet* 1995; 345:263.

352. Ballinger, A.B., Clark, M.L. "Severe acute hepatitis B infection after vaccination." *Lancet* 1994; 344:1292-1293.

353. Freed, G.L., et al. "Reactions of pediatricians to a new Centers for Disease Control recommendation for universal immunization of infants with hepatitis B vaccine." *Pediatrics* 1993; 91:699-702.

354. Freed, G.L., et al. "Family physician acceptance of universal hepatitis B immunization of infants." *Journal of Family Practice* 1993; 36: 153-157.

355. Dienstag, J.L., and Ryan, D.M. "Occupational exposure to hepatitis B virus in hospital personnel: infection or immunization?" *American Journal of Epidemiology* 1982; 115(1):26-39.

356. Classen, John Barthelow. "The Diabetes Epidemic and the Hepatitis B Vaccine." *New Zealand Medical Journal*. May 24, 1996, p. 366.

357. Classen, John Barthelow. "Childhood Immunisation and Diabetes Mellitus," *New Zealand Medical Journal*. May 24, 1996, p. 195.

358. Gross, K., et al. "Arthritis after hepatitis vaccination: report of three cases." *Scandinavian Journal of Rheumatology* 1995; 24:50-52.
359. Vautier, G., Carter, J.E. "Acute sero-positive rheumatoid arthritis occurring after hepatitis vaccination." *British Journal of Rheumatology* 1994; 33:991.
360. Lilic, D., Ghosh, S.K. "Liver dysfunction and DNA antibodies after hepatitis B vaccination." *Lancet* 1994; 344: pp. 1292-1293.
361. Poullin, P., Gabriel, B. "Thrombocytopenic purpura after recombinant hepatitis B vaccine." *Lancet* 1994; 334:1293.
362. Trevisani, F., et al. "Transverse myelitis following hepatitis B vaccination." *Journal of Hepatology* 1993; 19:317-318.
363. Morris, K., et al. "Nature and frequency of adverse reactions following hepatitis B vaccine injection in children in New Zealand, 1985-1988." Presented at the Vaccine Safety Committee, Institute of Medicine, Washington, DC, May 4, 1992.
364. Martinez, E., Domingo, P. "Evans's syndrome triggered by recombinant hepatitis B vaccine." *Clinical Infectious Diseases* 1992; 15:1051.
365. Herroelen, L., et al. "Central nervous system demyelination after immunization with recombinant hepatitis B vaccine." *Lancet* November 9, 1991; 338:1174-1175.
366. Hachulla, E., et al. "Reactive arthritis after hepatitis B vaccination." *Journal of Rheumatology* 1990; 17:1250-1251.
367. *Australian Adverse Drug Reactions Bulletin*, August 1990.
368. Shaw, F.E., Graham, D.J., et al. "Postmarketing surveillance for neurologic adverse events reported after hepatitis B vaccination." *American Journal of Epidemiology* 1988; 127(2):337-352.
369. Ribera, E.F., Dutka, A.J. "Polyneuropathy associated with administration of hepatitis B vaccine." *New England Journal of Medicine* 1983; 309:614-615.
370. See Notes 39 and 157.
371. Read the manufacturer's warnings on the hepatitis B vaccine package inserts.
372. See Note 262.
373. See Note 19, p. 246.
374. National Foundation for Infectious Diseases. "What Parents Need to Know About Chickenpox," (informational pamphlet). Bethesda, MD.
375. Preblud, S.R. "Varicella: complications and costs." *Pediatrics* 1986; 78:728-735.
376. See Note 7, p. 180. Also see Notes 374 and 375.
377. Halloran, M.E., et al. *American J of Epidemiology*, 1994; 140:81-104. As cited in *Medical Sciences Bulletin*, "Chickenpox vaccine approved." (April 1995), p. 2. www.pharminfo.com/pubs/msb/chipox.html
378. Lieu, T.A., et al. *Journal of the American Medical Association*, 1994; 271:375-381. As cited in *Time*, "Chicken Pox conundrum." (July 19, 1993), p. 53.
379. Watson, B.M., et al. "Modified chickenpox in children immunized with Oka-Merck varicella vaccine." *Pediatrics*, 1993; 91:17-22.
380. Naruse, H., et al. "Varicella infection complicated with meningitis after immunization." *Acta Paediatrica Japonica* 1993; 35:345-47.
381. American Academy of Pediatrics. "The chickenpox vaccine: What parents need to know" (public education brochure). p. 3. Reprinted online: www.aap.org/family/chckpox.htm
382. Wise, Robert P., et al. "Postlicensure safety surveillance for varicella vaccine." *Journal of the American Medical Association (JAMA)*, 284:10 (September 13, 2000), pp. 1271-79.
383. See Note 39.
384. See Note 382, p. 1278.
385. See Note 168, p. 45.
386. Salzman, M.B., et al. "Transmission of varicella-vaccine virus from a healthy 12-month-old child to his pregnant mother." *Journal of Pediatrics* (July 1997); 131(1 Pt 1):151-54.
387. See Note 382, p. 1277.
388. As noted on the chickenpox vaccine manufacturer's product labels.
389. As reported in an NVIC press release on the chickenpox vaccine, September 13, 2000. www.909shot.com/chickenpoxvaers91300.htm
390. See Note 382.
391. Ibid.
392. Ibid., p. 1273: Table 1.
393. Ibid., pp. 1274 and 1278.
394. Klinman, D., et al. *Nature Medicine* 2000; 6:381-82, 451-54.
395. McKinney, M. "Varicella zoster vaccine reactivates when immunity declines." *Reuters Health.* www.id.medscape.com/reuters/prof/2000/03/03.29/pb03290c.html
396. Plotkin, S. "Hell's fire and varicella-vaccine safety." *New England Journal of Medicine* 1988; 318:573-75.
397. Kohl, S., et al. "Natural varicella-zoster virus reactivation shortly after varicella immunization in a child." *Pediatric Infectious Disease Journal* 1999;18:1112-1113.
398. See Note 262.
399. Gellis, S. "Pediatric notes: The weekly commentary," Vol. 11:2 (January 15, 1987).
400. Broome, C.V. "Epidemiology of Haemophilus influenzae type b infection in the United States." *Pediatric Infectious Disease Journal* 1987; 6:779-82.
401. Mendelsohn, Robert S. "New vaccine to combat day care infections," *The People's Doctor Newsletter*, Vol. 9:11, p. 5. Figures reported by Dr. Stephen L. Coeni of the CDC.
402. Eskola, J. "Combined vaccination of Haemophilus influenzae type b conjugate and diphtheria-tetanus-pertussis containing acellular pertussis." *The Lancet Interactive*, Dec 11, 1999. www.findarticles.com/cf0/m0833/9195354/58184139/p1/article.jhtml
403. National Institutes of Health. "The haemophilus influenzae type b (Hib) vaccine—long-term

research pays off." www.niaid.nih.gov/publications/economic/vaccine.htm
404. Ibid.
405. "Updates: Vaccine Use Extended to Infants," _FDA Consumer_, January-February 1991: p. 2.
406. Centers for Disease Control and Prevention. "Frequently asked questions about Haemophilus influenzae type b (Hib) and Hib vaccine." www.cdc.gov/nip/Q&A/clinqa/hib.htm
407. Ibid.
408. See Note 403.
409. See Note 406.
410. Ibid.
411. Adams, W.G., et al. "Decline of childhood haemophilus influenzae type b (Hib) disease." _Journal of the American Medical Association_, 1993; 269:221-226.
412. Kaplan, S.L., et al. "Update on bacterial meningitis." _Journal of Child Neurology_, 1988; 3:82-93.
413. See Note 406.
414. Sell, S.H. "Haemophilus influenzae type b meningitis: manifestations and long-term sequelae." _Pediatric Infectious Disease Journal_ 1987; 6:775-778.
415. See Notes 406 and 411.
416. Smith, E., et al. "Changing incidence of haemophilus influenzae meningitis." _Pediatrics_, 1972; 50(5):723-727.
417. Bjune, G., et al. "Effect of outer membrane vesicle vaccine against group b meningococcal disease in Norway." _Lancet_, 1991; 338(8775):1093-1096.
418. See Note 168, p. 20.
419. Craighead, J. E. "Report of a workshop: disease accentuation after immunization with inactivated microbial vaccines." _Journal of Infectious Diseases_, 1975; 1312(6):749-54.
420. See Note 17. Authors of this study concluded that DPT injections are an important cause of "provocative disease."
421. Hinman, A., et al. "Immunization practices in developed countries." _Lancet_, 1990; 335:707-710.
422. Kimura, M., et al. "Acellular pertussis vaccines and fatal infections." _Lancet_, (April 16, 1988): 881-882.
423. See Note 210, pp. 132-133.
424. See Note 168, p. 21.
425. See Note 406.
426. Zwillich, Todd. "Hib rates in U.S. children higher among minorities than whites." _Reuters Medical News_, (August 18, 2000): www.id.medscape.com/reuters/prof/2000/08/08.18/20000818 epid003.html
427. See Note 406.
428. _Physician's Desk Reference_ (PDR); 53rd Edition. Medical Economics: Montvale, NJ. 1999, p. 3072.
429. See Note 426.
430. Ibid.
431. Mendelsohn, Robert. _But Doctor, About That Shot...The Risks of Immunizations and How to Avoid Them_, (Evanston, IL: The People's Doctor Newsletter, Inc., 1988), p. 88.
432. Weiss, R. "Meningitis Vaccine Stirs Controversy," _Science News_, Vol. 132; October 24, 1987, p. 260.
433. American Academy of Pediatrics. "Policy Statement: Haemophilus b polysaccharide vaccine (HbPV)," _AAP News_, (November 1987); p. 7.
434. Black, S., et al. "Efficacy of Haemophilus influenzae type b capsular polysaccharide vaccine," _Pediatric Infectious Disease Journal_, 1988; 7:149-156.
435. Harrison, L.H., et al. "A day care-based study of the efficacy of Haemophilus influenzae type b polysaccharide vaccine." _Journal of the American Medical Association_, 1988; 260:1413-1418.
436. Osterholm, M.T., et al. "Lack of efficacy of Haemophilus b polysaccharide vaccine in Minnesota." _Journal of the American Medical Association_, 1988; 260:1423-1428.
437. Shapiro, E.D., et al. "The protective efficacy of Haemophilus influenzae polysaccharide vaccine." _Journal of the American Medical Association_, 1988; 260:1419-1422.
438. Hiner, E.E., et al. "Spectrum of disease due to Haemophilus influenzae type b occurring in vaccinated children." _Journal of Infectious Disease_, 1988; 158(2):343-48.
439. Gellis, S.S. "Pediatric Notes: The Weekly Pediatric Commentary," Vol. 11:2 (January 15, 1987).
440. Daum, R.S. et al. "Decline in serum antibody to the capsule of Haemophilus influenzae type b in the immediate postimmunization period." _Journal of Pediatrics_, 1989; 1114:742-47.
441. Marchant, D.D., et al. "Depression of anticapsular antibody after immunization with Haemophilus influenzae type b polysaccharide-diphtheria conjugate vaccine." _Pediatric Infectious Disease Journal_, 1989; 320:75-81.
442. Sood, S.K., et al. "Disease caused by Haemophilus influenzae type b in the immediate period after homologous immunization: immunologic investigation." _Pediatrics_, 1990; 85 (4 Pt 2):698-704.
443. See Note 262.
444. See Notes 39 and 157.
445. See Note 428, pp. 1521.
446. Gervaix, M., et al. "Guillain-Barré syndrome following immunization with Haemophilus influenzae type b conjugate vaccine." _European Journal of Pediatrics_, 1993; 152: 613-14.
447. D'Cruz, O.F., et al. "Acute inflammatory demyelinating polyradiculoneuropathy (Guillain-Barré syndrome) after immunization with Haemophilus influenzae type b conjugate vaccine." _Journal of Pediatrics_, 1989; 115:743-46.
448. Vadheim, C.M., et al. "Effectiveness and safety of an Haemophilus influenzae type b conjugate vaccine (PRP-T) in young infants." _Pediatrics_, 1993; 92:272-79.
449. Ward, J., et al. "Efficacy of a Haemophilus influenzae type b conjugate vaccine in Alaska native infants." _New England Journal of Medicine_, 1990; 323(2):1393-1401.

450. Milstien, J.B., et al. "Adverse reactions reported following receipt of Haemophilus influenzae type b vaccine: an analysis after one year of marketing." *Pediatrics,* 1987; 80:270-74.

451. Granoff, D.M., et al. "Response to immunization with Haemophilus influenzae type b polysaccharide-pertussis vaccine and risk of haemophilus meningitis in children with the km(1) immunoglobulin allotype." *Journal of Clinical Investigation,* 1984; 74:1708-14.

452. Dokheel, T.M. "An epidemic of childhood diabetes in the United States." *Diabetes Care,* 1993; 16:1601-1611.

453. Gardner, S., et al. "Rising incidence of insulin dependent diabetes in children under 5 years in Oxford region: time trend analysis." *British Medical Journal,* 1997; 315:713-716.

454. Karvonen, M., et al. "Association between type 1 diabetes and Haemophilus influenzae type b vaccination: birth cohort study." *British Medical Journal,* 1999; 318:1169-1172.

455. Classen, J.B., et al. "Haemophilus vaccine study in Finland supports a relationship between vaccines and diabetes." www.vaccines.net/newpage16.htm

456. Classen, J.B., et al. "Association between type 1 diabetes and Hib vaccine." *British Medical Journal,* 1999; 319:1133.

457. PRNewswire. "Hemophilus meningitis vaccine linked to diabetes increase; many diabetics may be eligible for compensation." May 7, 1999. www.islet.org/forum011/messages/7958.htm

458. See Note 456.

459. See Note 457.

460. Ibid.

461. See Notes 456 and 457.

462. See Note 456.

463. Classen, J.B. "Public should be told that vaccines may have long term adverse effects." *British Medical Journal,* 1999; 318:193.

464. See Note 456.

465. See Note 262.

466. As noted on the inserts from the vaccine manufacturer (clinical pharmacology). www.pneumo.com/vaccine/PI.html

467. See Note 428, pp. 1524 and 1861.

468. Ibid., P. 1534.

469. Iannelli, V.R. "Pneumococcus (Prevnar)." *Keepkidshealthy.com* (August 27, 2000). www.keepkidshealthy.com/welcome/immunizations/ pneumococcus.html

470. Forrester, H.L., et al. "Inefficacy of pneumococcal vaccine in a high-risk population." *American Journal of Medicine,* 1987; 83:425-30.

471. Simberkoff, M.S., et al. "Efficacy of pneumococcal vaccine in high-risk patients: results of a Veterans Administration cooperative study." *New England Journal of Medicine,* 1986; 315:1318-27.

472. "Pneumococcal vaccines ineffective." *Utah Vaccine Awareness Coalition,* December 2000, Vol.2, No. 3., p. 6.

473. See Note 469.

474. See Note 466.

475. "AAP recommends pneumococcal vaccine for children younger than age 2." *Medscape Wire* (June 9, 2000). www.id.medscape.com/MedscapeWire/2000/0600/medwire.0609.AAP.html

476. Red Book Report of the Committee on Infectious Diseases, 23rd edition. *American Academy of Pediatrics,* 1994: 371.

477. Black, S., Shinefield, H., et al. "Efficacy, safety and immunogenicity of heptavalent pneumococcal conjugate vaccine in children." Northern California Kaiser Permanente Vaccine Study Center Group. *Pediatric Infectious Disease Journal,* March 2000;19(3):187-95.

478. Black, S., Shinefield, H., et al. "Efficacy of heptavalent conjugate pneumococcal vaccine (Lederle Laboratories) in 37,000 infants and children." Results of the Northern California Kaiser Permanente Efficacy Trial. 36th ICAAC, San Diego, CA. September 24-27, 1998.

479. See Note 466 (warnings). www.pneumo.com/vaccine/PI.html

480. Overturf, G. "Technical report: prevention of pneumococcal infections, including the use of pneumococcal conjugate and polysaccharide vaccines and antibiotic prophylaxix (RE9960)." *American Academy of Pediatrics and the Committee on Infectious Diseases.* wwwaap.org/policy/re9960t.html

481. See Note 466 (adverse reactions). www.pneumo.com/vaccine/PI.html

482. See Note 262.

483. Department of Health and the Health Education Authority. "Meningococcal C vaccine (Meningitis C) factsheet." 1999, p. 1. British.

484. See Note 428, p. 2339.

485. Replacement chapter for "Immunisation against infectious disease" 1996: Chapter 23, Meningococcal. [British] Department of Health. (Published by the NHS Executive.) www.doh.gov.uk/meningitis-vaccine/chapter23.htm

486. Ibid.

487. Communicable Disease Surveillance and Response. Meningococcal Disease Update: 1998 Cases and Deaths of Meningococcal Disease, Reported to WHO. *WHO/OMS,* 1998. (Last updated July 11, 2000). www.who.int/emc/diseases/meningitis/1998meningtable.html

488. PR Newswire. "North American Vaccine accelerates timeline for seeking approval for meningitis vaccine." April 12, 1999. www.findarticles.com/ m4PRN/1999_April_12/54341659/p1/article.jhtml

489. Varnell, M. "CDC recommends college students get meningococcal vaccine." *Reuter's Medical News,* July 3, 2000.

490. See Note 483.

491. "The new Meningitis C vaccine." [British] Department of Health. (Published by the NHS Executive.) www.doh.gov.uk/meningitis-vaccine/newcvaccine.htm

492. Woodman, R. "Meningitis C vaccine not responsible for deaths." *Reuters Medical News,* September 5, 2000.

493. Ibid.

494. See Note 428, p. 2339 and Note 485.

495. "Frequently asked questions about meningitis." [British] Department of Health. (Published by Health Promotion England.) www.immunisation.org.uk/menfaqs.html

496. Ibid.

497. See Note 262.

498. Meningococcal disease and college students. *MMWR Morb Mortal Wkly Rep.* 2000; 49(RR-7):13-20.

499. Steele, R.W. "Pediatric ID Update: The HUS-Antibiotic Connection, and Vaccine News." (Meningococcal Vaccine for College Students.) *Medscape Infectious Diseases,* 2000.

500. Ibid.

501. CDC. "Prevention of hepatitis A through active or passive immunization: recommendations of the Advisory Committee on Immunization Practices (ACIP)." *MMWR Weekly* (October 1, 1999); 48(RR12):1-37.

502. Merck Data Sheet. "Hepatitis A." Merck & Co. www.merck.com/disease/preventable/hepa

503. See Note 501.

504. Department of Human Services, Australia. "Hepatitis A: the facts." www.hna.ffh.vic.gov.au/phb/9911053/index.htm

505. See Note 501.

506. Ibid.

507. Winkler, D. "Hepatitis A facts." *Concerned Parents for Vaccine Safety.* www.access1.net/via/vaccine/hepafacts.htm

508. See Notes 501, 502, and 504.

509. See Note 501.

510. See Notes 501 and 507.

511. SmithKline Beecham Biologicals, unpublished data, 1995. As cited in Note 501.

512. See Notes 39 and 501.

513. See Note 502.

514. See Note 501.

515. CDC. "Respiratory syncytial virus." National Center for Infectious Disease, 1999. www.cdc.gov/ncidod/dvrd/nrevss/rsvfeat.htm

516. Public Health Laboratory Service, United Kingdom. "Seasonal diseases: respiratory syncytial virus (RSV) infections." www.phls.co.uk/seasonal/rsv/RSV13.htm (March 16, 2000.)

517. Baltimore, J.G. "RSV—a serious subject." *The Triplet Connection,* 2000. www.triplet connection.com/rsv_new.html

518. See Note 515.

519. Ibid.

520. See Note 517.

521. Travel and Health. "Questions and answers on Synagis." www. travelandhealth.com/synagis.htm

522. Applied Genetic News. "Eat your vaccine, dear." *Business Communications Company* (August 2000). www.findarticles.com/cf_dls/m0DED/1_21/65016226/p1/article.jhtml

523. See Note 517.

524. FDA. "FDA licenses biotech product to prevent serious RSV disease." *U.S. Department of Health and Human Services* (June 19, 1998). www.fda.gov/bbs/topics/answers/ans00878.html

525. Package Inserts. "Synagis®" (Palivizumab) for intramuscular administration." *Medimmune, Inc.,* 1999. www.medimmune.com/products/htmlpis/synagispi.html

526. Morris, J.A., et al. "Recovery of cytopathogenic agent from chimpanzees with coryza (22538)." *Proc Soc Exp Biol Med* 1956; 92:544-49.

527. See Note 210, p. 153.

528. Ibid.

529. Parrot, R.H., et al. "II. Serological studies over a 34-month period in children with bronchiolitis, pneumonia and minor respiratory diseases." *Journal of the American Medical Association* 1961; 176(8):653-57.

530. Chanock, R.M., et al. "Respiratory syncytial virus." *Journal of the American Medical Association* 1961; 176(8):647-53.

531. Ibid.

532. Hamparian, V., et al. "Recovery of new viruses (coryza) from cases of common cold in human adults." *Proc Soc Exp Med Biol* 1961; 108:444-453.

533. Keep Kids Healthy. "Preventing RSV." www.keepkidshealthy.com/welcome/infections guide/preventing_rsv.html (2002.)

534. Ibid.

535. "More on cost of synagis..." (Posted March 26, 1999 on an internet forum.) www.home.vicnet. net.au/~garyh/preemie_forum/old-messages/4799.html

536. The Impact RSV Study Group. "Palivizumab, a humanized respiratory syncytial virus monoclonal antibody, reduces hospitalization from respiratory syncytial virus infection in high-risk infants." *Pediatrics* 1998; 102:531-537.

537. See Note 525.

538. See Notes 525 and 536.

539. Ibid.

540. Ibid.

541. Ibid.

542. Tant, Carl. *Awesome Green* (Angleton, TX: Biotech Publications, 1994), pp. 108-115.

543. See Congressional Bill, H.R. 78, 103rd Congress, 1st Session (January 5, 1993).

544. Moskowitz, R. "Vaccination: A Sacrament of Modern Medicine," *Mothering* (Spring 1992), p. 53.

545. Leviton, R. "A Shot in the Dark," *Yoga Journal* (May/June, 1992), p. 128.
546. Turkington, C.A. "Anthrax." *Gale Encyclopedia of Medicine* 1999. www.findarticles.com/cf_dls/g2601/0000/2601000086/print.jhtml
547. "Anthrax." Encarta Encyclopedia (accessed October 2001). www.encarta.msn.com/find/Concise.asp?z=1&pg=2&ti=761577286
548. CDC. "Anthrax." (Accessed October 2001); www.cdc.gov/ncidod/dbmd/diseaseinfo/anthrax_g.htm
549. Shlyakov, E.N., et al. "Human live anthrax vaccine in the former USSR." *Vaccine* 1994; 12: 727.
550. Turnbull, P.C.B. "Anthrax vaccines; past, present and future." *Vaccine* 1991; 9:533.
551. Ibid.
552. Anthony, B.F., et al. "The role of the FDA in vaccine testing and licensure." In Lelvine, M.M., et al., (eds.): New Generation Vaccines, ed. 2. (New York, NY: Marcel Dekker, 1997), p. 1185.
553. See Note 548.
554. Ritter, M. "Precautions on ranches and in factories have helped keep the disease rare in the U.S." *Albuquerque Journal* (October 21, 2001), p. B8.
555. Stolberg, S.G., et al. "After a week of reassurances, Ridge's anthrax message is grim." *The New York Times* (October 26,2001). www.nytimes.com
556. See Notes 546 and 548.
557. Ibid.
558. Flegel, D.E. "FDA oks use of doxycycline after anthrax exposure." *WebMD* (October 22,2001). www.content.health.msn.com/content/article/4048.114
559. "Cipro." *Drug InfoNet* 2000. www.druginfonet.com/cipro.htm
560. CDC. *MMWR Morb Mortal Wkly Rep* 2001; 50:1031-1034.
561. Reuters Medical News. "Postal workers report high rate of adverse events from anthrax prophylaxis." *Medscape*, (November 29, 2001).
562. Park, A. "Cipro to Doxy: Why the Switch?" *Time.com* (November 5, 2001). www.time.com/time/magazine/printout/0,8816,181572,00.html
563. Health Square. "Doryx (Doxycycline hyclate)." *The PDR Family Guide to Prescription Drugs*. www.healthsquare.com/rx/doryx.htm (Accessed 11/1/01)
564. Begley, S., et al. "Anthrax: what you need to know." *Newsweek* (October 29, 2001), p. 39.
565. See notes 546 and 548.
566. Ibid.
567. Ibid.
568. See note 564.
569. See Notes 546 and 548.
570. Brachman, P.S., et al. "Field evaluation of a human anthrax vaccine." *American Journal of Public Health* 1962; 52:632-645.
571. Ibid.
572. Nass, M. "New vaccines and new vaccine technology: anthrax vaccine—model of a response to the biologic warfare threat." *Infectious Disease Clinics of North America* (W.B. Saunders Company) 1999; 13(1):189.
573. Institute of Medicine. "An Assessment of the Safety of the Anthrax Vaccine." (March 30, 2000), pp. 3-4.
574. Ibid.
575. Official Document. "Anthrax vaccine chronology." *JFSorg*, 2001. www.enter.net/~jfsorg/timeline.pdf
576. Ibid.
577. Ivins, B.E., et al. "Immunization studies with attenuated strains of Bacillus anthracis." *Infect Immun* 1986; 52:454.
578. Little, S.F., et al. "Comparative efficacy of Bacillus anthracis live spore vaccine and protective antigen vaccine against anthrax in the guinea pig." *Infect Immun* 1986; 52:509-512
579. Ivins, B.E., et al. "Recent advances in the development of an improved, human anthrax vaccine." *European Journal of Epidemiology* 1988; 4:12.
580. Turnbull, P.C.B., et al. "Antibodies to anthrax toxin in humans and guinea pigs and their relevance to protective immunity." *Med Microbiol Immunol* 1988; 177:293.
581. Ivins, B.E., et al. "Immunization against anthrax with aromatic compound-dependent (Aromutants) of Bacillus anthracis and with recombinant strains of Bacillus subtilis that produce anthrax protective antigen." *Infect Immun* 1990; 58:303.
582. Ivins, B.E., et al. "Immunization against anthrax with Bacillus anthracis protective antigen combined with adjuvants." *Infect Immun* 1992; 60:662.
583. Ivins, B.E., et al. "Efficacy of a standard human anthrax vaccine against Bacillus anthracis spore challenge in guinea pigs." *Vaccine* 1994; 12:872.
584. Ivins, B.E., et al. "Experimental anthrax vaccines: efficacy of adjuvants combined with protective antigen against aerosol Bacillus anthracis spore challenge in guinea pigs." *Vaccine* 1995; 13:1779.
585. Welkos, S.L., et al. "Comparative safety and efficacy against Bacillus anthracis of protective antigen and live vaccines in mice." *Microb Pathog* 1988; 5:127.
586. Welkos, S.L., et al. "Pathogenesis and host resistance to Bacillus anthracis: a mouse model." *Salisbury Medical Bulletin* 1990; 68:49.
587. See Notes 581 and 582.
588. Friedlander, A.M., et al. "Postexposure prophylaxis against experimental inhalation anthrax." *Journal of Infectious Diseases* 1993; 167:1239.
589. Ivins, B.E., et al. "Efficacy of a standard human anthrax vaccine against Bacillus anthracis aerosol spore challenge in rhesus monkeys." *Salisbury Medical Bulletin* (Special Supplement) 1996; 87:125-126.

590. Enserink, M. "This time it was real: knowledge of anthrax put to the test." *Science* 2001; 294: 490-91.

591. See Note 589.

592. Ibid.

593. Ivins, B.E., et al. "Comparative efficacy of experimental anthrax vaccine candidates against inhalation anthrax in rhesus macaques." *Vaccine* 1998; 16, No. 11/12:1141-1148.

594. Ibid.

595. Fellows, P., et al. "Anthrax vaccine efficacy against B. anthracis strains of diverse geographic origin." Presented at the International Anthrax Conference (September 1998). As noted in the Congressional testimony of Dr. Meryl Nass: *Subcommittee on National Security, Veterans Affairs and International Relations* (April 29, 1999).

596. Zuckerman, Diana, PhD., and Olson, Patricia, D.V.M., Ph.D., "Is Military Research Hazardous to Veterans' Health? Lessons from the Persian Gulf: Preliminary Staff Findings," *United States Senate, Committee on Veterans' Affairs* (May 6, 1994).

597. France, D. "The families who are dying for our country." *Redbook* (September 1994), p. 116.

598. "Experts find link to war illness." *The Albuquerque Tribune* (April 10, 1995), pp. A1+.

599. Majority Staff. "Unproven Force Protection." *Subcommittee on National Security, Veterans Affairs and International relations, House Committee on Government Reform.* (February 17, 2000), p. 6.

600. Oversight of the Anthrax Vaccine Inoculation Program (March 24, 1999); Anthrax: Safety and Efficacy of the Mandatory Vaccine (April 29, 1999); Oversight of DoD Sole Source Anthrax Vaccine Procurement (June 30, 1999); Anthrax Vaccine Adverse Reactions (July 21, 1999); Impact of the Anthrax Vaccine Program on Reserve and National Guard Units (September 29, 1999); Anthrax Vaccine Immunization Program: What Have We Learned? (October 3,10, 2000). *Government Reform Committee Hearings,* Washington, DC.

601. In an unpublished "Fort Bragg" Department of Defense Study: Final Report to the FDA. As cited by Meryl Nass in a Hearing on Anthrax Vaccine Safety, *Committee on Government Reform* (April 29, 1999).

602. Testimony in a hearing on Anthrax Vaccine Safety (April 29, 1999).

603. Ibid.

604. See Note 2, Volume 17, p. 513.

605. WebMD. "What is smallpox?" 2001. www.content.health.msn.com/printing/article/4058.261

606. *Microsoft Encarta Online Encyclopedia,* "Smallpox." (October 26, 2001). www.encarta.msn.com

607. Seercom. "Smallpox: Treatment." www.seercom.com/bluto/smallpox/treatment.html

608. White, W. *The Story of a Great Delusion.* (London: E.W. Allen, 1885), p. xviii.

609. Cohen, J., et al. "Vaccines for biodefense: a system in distress," *Science* (October 19, 2001), p. 499.

610. Rosenthal, S.R., et al. "Developing new smallpox vaccines." *Emerging Infectious Diseases, CDC;* 7(6), Nov-Dec, 2001.

611. Stolberg, S.G. "Immunization: vast uncertainty on smallpox vaccine." *New York Times* (October 19, 2001). www.nytimes.com/2001/10/19/national/19SMAL.html

612. Orent, W. "The smallpox wars: biowarfare vs. public health." *The American Prospect* 1999; 10(44).

613. Barquet, N., et al. "Smallpox: The triumph over the most terrible of the ministers of death." *Annals of Internal Medicine* (October 15, 1997); 127:635-642.

614. Edwardes, E.J. *A Concise History of Small-pox and Vaccination in Europe.* (London: H.K. Lewis, 1902).

615. Fenner, F. "Nature, nurture and my experience with smallpox eradication." *eMJA* 1999; 171:638+. www.mja.com.au/public/issues/171_11_061299/fenner/fenner.html

616. WHO. "Fifty Years of the World Health Organization in the Western Pacific Region—Report of the Regional Director to the Regional Committee for the Western Pacific: Chapter 27, Smallpox." www.who.org.ph/public/policy/50TH/Ch_27.html

617. As documented by the CDC and World Health Organization.

618. Tandy, E.C. "The regulation of nuisances in the American Colonies." *American Journal of Public Health* (October 1923); 13(10):810-813.

619. Chase, A. *Magic Shots: A Human and Scientific Account of the Long and Continuing Struggle to Eradicate Infectious Diseases by Vaccination.* (NY: William Morrow and Co., 1982).

620. Bayne-Jones, S. *The Evolution of Preventive Medicine in the United States Army, 1607-1939* (Washington, DC: Office of the Surgeon General, Dept. of the Army, 1968), p. 21.

621. See Note 23, p. 12.

622. Parish, H.J. *A History of Immunization,* (Edinburgh: E & S Livingstone, 1965).

623. See Note 23, p. 33.

624. Shelton, H.M. *Vaccine and Serum Evils* (San Antonio, Texas: Health Research, 1966), p. 23. Citing official statistics from England.

625. See Note 24, p. 32.

626. See Note 23, p. 27.

627. Ibid., p. 13.

628. Ibid.

629. Koren, T. "Tedd Koren's 2nd November 2001 newsletter," *Koren Publications, Inc.* (November 9, 2001).

630. Ibid.

631. See Note 23, p. 16.

632. "Vaccination in Italy," *New York Medical Journal* (July 22, 1899).

633. Ibid.

634. See Note 624, pp. 20-21.

635. Ibid., pp. 21-22.
636. See Note 24, p. 36.
637. Ibid., p. 22.
638. Ibid., pp. 23-24. Citing official statistics from England and Wales.
639. See Note 608, p. xxi.
640. See Note 24, pp. 36-37.
641. See Note 629.
642. *New York Press* (January 26, 1909).
643. See Note 23, pp. 21-24; 42, 72.
644. Garrow, R.P. "Fatality rates of small-pox in the vaccinated and unvaccinated," *British Medical Journal* (January 14, 1928), p. 74.
645. Parry, L.A. "Fatality rates of small-pox in the vaccinated and unvaccinated," *British Medical Journal* (January 21, 1928), p. 116.
646. In a congressional statement by Senator Dolliver, United States Senate (February 25, 1909).
647. United States Department of Agriculture. *Farmer's Bulletin* (April 22, 1915), p. 15.
648. *Journal of the American Medical Association* (July 1926).
649. *Lancet* (September 4, 1926).
650. *Lancet* (October 9, 1926).
651. Garrow, R.P. "Fatality rates of small-pox in the vaccinated and unvaccinated," *British Medical Journal* (January 14, 1928), p. 74.
652. See Note 645.
653. DeVries, E. *Postvaccinal Perivenous Encephalitis* (Amsterdam: Elsevier Publishing Company, 1959).
654. Dick, G.W.A. "Scientific Proceedings; Symposium on Virus Diseases. 13th Annual Meeting of the British Medical Association, Belfast." *British Medical Journal*, 1962; 2:319.
655. Dixon, C.W. *Smallpox, London* (J & A Churchill, Ltd., 1962).
656. Spillane, J.D., et al. "The neurology of Jennerian vaccination—a clinical account of the neurological complications which occurred during the smallpox epidemic in South Wales in 1962." *Brain,* 1964; 87:1-44.
657. Miller, H., et al. "Multiple sclerosis and vaccination." *British Medical Journal,* (April 22, 1967), pp. 210-213.
658. Neff, J.M., et al. "Complications of smallpox vaccination, United States, 1963. II. Results obtained by four statewide surveys." *Pediatrics,* 1967; 39:916-923.
659. Lane, M.J. "Complications of smallpox vaccination," *New England Journal of Medicine,* 1968; 281(22):1201-1208.
660. Redfield, R., et al. "Disseminated vaccinia in a military recruit with human immunodeficiency virus (HIV) disease." *New England Journal of Medicine* (March 12, 1987), p. 673.
661. Wright, P. "Smallpox vaccine 'triggered AIDS virus.'" *London Times,* (May 11, 1987).
662. Rappoport, J. "Smallpox vaccine as AIDS trigger." *L. A. Weekly,* (June 5-11, 1987), p. 8.
663. See Note 661.
664. Franks, G. *AIDS and Vaccinations: The London Times Reports.* (Denton, TX: Pure Water Products, 1988), pp. 21-23.
665. See Note 661.
666. Ibid.
667. Ibid.
668. Bazell, R., et al. "Anthrax fears close Senate offices." *MSNBC* (October 16, 2001). www.msnbc.com/news/638169.asp?pne=msn
669. Associated Press. "Congress closes for anthrax sweep." *The Santa Fe New Mexican* (October 18, 2001), p. A1.
670. Bazell, R., et al. "Anthrax strains in 3 attacks linked." *MSNBC* (October 19, 2001). www.msnbc.com/news/638169.asp?pne=msn
671. Check, E., et al. "Bioterrorism: bracing for the worst." *Newsweek* (October 29, 2001), p. 41.
672. Center for Strategic and International Studies. "Dark Winter: A Bioterrorism Exercise." *Johns Hopkins Center for Civilian Biodefense Studies; Anser Institute for Homeland Security,* (June 2001). www.hopkins-biodefense.org
673. Ibid.
674. Meltzer, M.I., et al. "Modeling potential responses to smallpox as a bioterrorist weapon—Appendix I: A mathematical review of the transmission of smallpox." *Emerging Infectious Diseases, CDC;* 7(6), Nov-Dec, 2001.
675. Milloy, S. "Smallpox attack exaggerated." *Fox News* (October 5, 2001). www.foxnews.com/story/0,2933,35758,00.html
676. Miller, J., et al. "September 11 attacks led to push for more smallpox vaccine." *The New York Times* (October 22, 2001).
677. See Note 609.
678. Radio National. "The Health Report: Monkeypox." *Australian Broadcasting Corporation* (September 1, 1997).
679. Stolberg, S.G. "Immunization: Vast Uncertainty on smallpox vaccine." *New York Times* (October 19, 2001). www.nytimes.com/2001/10/19/national/19SMAL.html
680. See Note 609, p. 500.
681. Miller, J. "U.S. set to retain smallpox stocks." *The New York Times* (November 16, 2001).
682. Gostin, L.O. "The Model State Emergency Health Powers Act." Prepared by The Center for Law and the Public's Health at Georgetown and Johns Hopkins Universities for the Centers for Disease Control and Prevention. (As of October 23, 2001), pp. 1-40. www.publichealthlaw.net
683. Ibid., pp. 28-29.
684. Ibid., pp. 16-18; Sections 303: Effect of Declaration, and 304: Enforcement.
685. Knight Ridder Newspapers. "Health agency proposes quarantine plan for states." *The Santa*

Fe New Mexican, p. A1+.
686. See Note 682, p. 39; Section 807: Repeals.
687. See Note 682.
688. Keep Kids Healthy. Influenza. www.keepkidshealthy.com/schoolage/schoolageproblems/influenza.html p. 1.
689. Centers for Disease Control and Prevention (CDC). "Vaccine Information: Influenza Vaccine." www.cdc.gov/ncidod/diseases/flu/fluvac.htm pp. 3-4.
690. World Health Organization (WHO) Press Release. "Experts decide content of 1999-2000 Northern Hemisphere influenza vaccine." February 17, 1999.
691. See Note 428, pp. 2324 and 3315.
692. Connaught Laboratories. "The Making of a Flu Vaccine." Los Angeles Times (Reprinted in the Kansas City Star), February 24, 1993.
693. Ibid.
694. National Vaccine Information Center (NVIC). "The Flu and the Flu Vaccine." www.909shot.com/flufax.htm
695. See Note 689, p. 2.
696. Hurwitz, E.S., et al. "Guillain-Barré syndrome and the 1978-79 influenza vaccine." New England J of Med. 1981; 304:1557-61.
697. Kaplan, J.E., et al. "Guillain-Barré syndrome in the United States, 1978-1981: Additional observation from the national surveillance system." Neurology. 33:633-37.
698. Scheibner, V. "Flu vaccination: Is it safe?" Natural Health (June/July 1993), pp. 19-21.
699. See Note 689, pp. 2-3 and Note 694.
700. See Note 694.
701. Lohse, A., et al. "Vascular purpura and cryoglobulinemia after influenza vaccination. Case-report and literature review." Rev Rhum Engl Ed. 1999 June; 66(6):359-60.
702. Schmutz, J.L., et al. "Does influenza vaccination induce bullous pemphigoid?" Ann Dermatol Vernereol. 1999 Oct;126(10):765. [French]
703. Cummins, D., et al. "Haematological changes associated with influenza vaccination in people aged over 65: case report and prospective study." Clin Lab Haematol. 1998 Oct; 20(5):285-7.
704. Downs, A.M., et al. "Does influenza vaccination induce bullous pemphigoid? A report of four cases." Br J Dermatol. 1998 Feb;138(2):363.
705. Kawasaki, A., et al. "Bilateral anterior ischemic optic neuropathy following influenza vaccination." J Neuroophthalmol. 1998 March; 18(1):56-9.
706. Lasky, T., et al. "The Guillain-Barré syndrome and the 1992-1993 and 1993-1994 influenza vaccines." N Engl J Med. 1998 Dec 17; 339(25):1797-802.
707. Park, C.L., et al. "Does influenza vaccination exacerbate asthma?" Drug Saf. 1998 Aug;19(2):83-88.
708. Ramakrishnan, N., et al. "Thrombotic thrombocytopenic purpura following influenza vaccination—a brief case report." Conn Med. 1998 Oct; 62(10):587-8.
709. Selvaraj, N., et al. "Hemiparesis following influenza vaccination." Postgrad Med J. 1998 Oct; 74(876):633-5.
710. Confino, I., et al. "Erythromelalgia following influenza vaccine in a child." Clin Exp Rheumatol. 1997 Jan-Feb;15(1):111-3.
711. Desson, J.F. et al. "Acute benign pericarditis after anti-influenza vaccination." Presse Med. 1997 Mar 22; 26(9):415. [French]
712. Hull, T.P., et al. "Optic neuritis after influenza vaccination." Am J Ophthalmol. 1997 Nov; 124(5):703-4.
713. Kelsall, J.T., et al. "Microscopic polyangiitis after influenza vaccination." J Rheumatol. 1997 Jun; 24(6):1198-202.
714. Owensby J.E., et al. "Cellulitis and myositis caused by agrobacterium radiobacter and Haemophilus parainfluenzae after influenza virus vaccination." South Med J. 1997 Jul; 90(7):752-4.
715. Bernad Valles, M., et al. "Adverse reactions to different types of influenza vaccines." Med Clin (Barc). 1996 Jan 13;106(1):11-4. [Spanish]
716. Fournier, B., et al. "Bullous pemphigoid induced by vaccination." Br J Dermatol. 1996 Jul;135(1):153-4.
717. Honkanen, P.O., et al. "Reactions following administration of influenza vaccine along or with pneumococcal vaccine to the elderly." Arch Intern Med. 1996 Jan 22;156(2):205-8.
718. Lear, J.T., et al. "Bullous pemphigoid following influenza vaccination." Clin Exp Dermatol. 1996 Sep; 21(5):392.
719. Ray, C.L., et al. "Bilateral optic neuropathy associated with influenza vaccination." J Neuroophthalmol. 1996 Sep; 16(3):182-4.
720. Antony, S.J., et al. "Postvaccinial (influenza) disseminated encephalopathy (Brown-Sequard syndrome)." J Natl Med Assoc. 1995 Sep; 87(9):705-8.
721. Cambiaghi. S., et al. "Gianotti-Crosti syndrome in an adult after influenza virus vaccination." Dermatology. 1995;191(4):340-1.
722. Herderschee, D., et al. "Myelopathy following influenza vaccination." Ned Tijdschr Geneeskd. 1995 Oct 21;139(42):2152-4. [Dutch]
723. Biasi, D., et al. "A case of reactive arthritis after influenza after influenza vaccination." Clin Rheumatol. 1994 Dec;13(4)645.
724. Blanche, P., et al. "Development of uveitis following vaccination for influenza." Clin Infect Dis. 1994 Nov;19(5):979.
725. Bodokh, I., et al. "Reactivation of bullous pemphigoid after influenza vaccination." Therapie. 1994 Mar-Apr; 49(2):154. [French]
726. Brown, M.A., et al. "Rheumatic complications of influenza vaccination." Aust N Z J Med. 1994 Oct; 24(5):572-3.
727. Beijer, W.E., et al. "Polymyalgia rheumatica and influenza vaccination." Dtsch Med

Wochenschr. 1993 Feb 5;118(5):164-5. [German]

728. Boutros, N., et al. "Delirium following influenza vaccination." *Am J Psychiatry.* 1993 Dec; 150(12):1899.

729. Mader, R., et al. "Systemic vasculitis following influenza vaccination—report of 3 cases and literature review." *J Rheumatol.* 1993 Aug; 20(8):1429-31. Review.

730. Robinson, T., et al. "Side effects of influenza vaccination." *Br J Gen Pract.* 1992 Nov; 42(364):489-90.

731. Ward, D.L., Re: "Guillian-Barré syndrome and influenza vaccination in the US Army, 1980-1988." *Am J Epidemiol.* 1992 Aug 1;136(3):374-6.

732. Young, G.. "Side effects of influenza immunization." *Br J Gen Pract.* 1992 Mar; 42(356):131.

733. Roscelli, J.D., et al. "Guillain-Barré syndrome and influenza vaccination in the US Army, 1980-1988." *Am J Epidemiol.* 1991 May 1; 133(9):952-5.

734. Molina, M., et al. "Leukocytoclastic vasculitis secondary to flu vaccination." *Med Clin (Barc).* 1990 Jun 9; 95(2):78. [Spanish]

735. Pelosio, A., et al. "Influenza vaccination and polyradiculoneuritis of the Guillain-Barré type." *Medicina (Firenze).* 1990 Apr-Jun;10(2):169. [Italian]

736. Buchner, H., et al. "Polyneuritis cranialis? Brain stem encephalitis and myelitis following preventive influenza vaccination." *Nervenarzt.* 1988 Nov; 59(11):679-82. [German]

737. See Note 262.

738. See Note 689, p. 1.

739. Ibid.

740. Ibid.

741. Advisory Committee on Immunization Practices. Prevention and Control of Influenza, Pt. I: Vaccine Recommendations of the ACIP. *MMWR Morb Mortal Wkly Rep,* 1993;42 (RR-6):1-13.

742. Brammer, T.L. "Surveillance for Influenza—United States: 1994-95, 1995-96, and 1996-97 Seasons." *Morbidity and Mortality Weekly Report: CDC.* April 28, 2000. Also See Note 9.

743. See Note 689, pp. 1-2, and Note 694.

744. Fox, M. "Study: Giving Flu Vaccine Doesn't Save Money." *Reuters.* www.dailynews.yahoo.com/h/nm/ 20001003/sc/health_flu_dc_3.html p. 1.

745. See Note 742.

746. Norton, A. "Flu shots cuts misery, but not costs." *Reuters.* www.dailynews.yahoo.com/h/nm/20001004/hl/ flu_shots_1.html

747. *Morbidity and Mortality Weekly Report: CDC.* 2004; 53:8-11.

748. Stein, R. "Flu season may be severe." *Washingtonpost.com.* Nov. 18, 2003. www.washington post.com/wp-dyn/articles/A54059-2003Nov17.html Also see NVIC Press Release, Dec. 10, 2003.

749. See Note 689, pp. 3 and 7.

750. Alling, D.W., et al. "A study of excess mortality during influenza epidemics in the US: 1968-1976." *Am J Epidemiol.* 1981; 113:30-43.

751. Eickhoff, T.C., et al. "Observations of excess mortality associated with epidemic influenza." *JAMA.* 1961; 176:776-782.

752. See Note 741.

753. Kuhle, C. L., et al. "An Influenza Outbreak in an Immunized Nursing Home Population: Inadequate Host Response or Vaccine Failure?" *Annals of Long-Term Care,* 1998; 6[3]:72.

754. Clarke, T. "Nasal flu vaccine approved." *MMCAP.* June 18, 2003.

755. Tucker, M. "Flu shot backed for ages 6-23 months." *Family Practice News.* November 15, 2003.

756. Advisory Committee on Immunization Practices. Prevention and Control of Influenza: Recommendations of the ACIP. *MMWR Morb Mortal Wkly Rep,* 1996; 45:1-24.

757. See Note 262.

758. See Notes 741, 750, 751, and 753.

759. Woodman, Richard. "UK offers free flu vaccinations to elderly, but millions might not take advantage." *Reuters Medical News,* September 26, 2000.

760. Recer, Paul. "Study: health workers major sources of flu in old-age homes." *Associated Press,* October 9, 1997. www.s-t.com/daily/10-97/10-09-97/a06wn032.htm

761. See Note 262.

762. Moskowitz, R. "Immunizations: A Dissenting View," In *Dissent in Medicine—Nine Doctors Speak Out* (Contemporary Books, 1985), pp. 133-166.

763. See Note 10, pp. 33-34.

764. Buttram, H.E. and Hoffman, J.C. *Vaccinations and Immune Malfunctions,* (Humanitarian Publishing Co., 1982), p. 47.

. 765. James, W. *Immunization: The Reality Behind the Myth,* (Bergin & Garvey, 1988), pp. 14-15.

766. Kalokerinos, A. and Dettman. "A Supportive Submission," *The Dangers of Immunisation.* (Warburton, Victoria, Australia: Biological Research Institute, 1979), p. 49.

767. See Note 143, p. 32.

768. Ibid.

769. Moskowitz, R. *The Case Against Immunizations,* (Washington, DC: The National Center for Homeopathy, 1983), p. 15.

770. See Note 765, pp. 15-16.

771. Ibid., pp. 16-17.

772. *World Medicine,* (London: Clareville House, September 22, 1971), pp. 69-72.

773. See Note 765, p. 10.

774. Buttram, H. "Live Virus Vaccines and Genetic Mutation," *Hlth. Consc.,* (Apr 1990), pp. 44-45.

775. Blanck, G., et al. "Multiple Insertions and Tandem Repeats of Origin-Mins Simian Virus 40 DNA in Transformed Rat and Mouse Cells." *Journal of Virology,* (May 1988), pp. 1520-1523.

776. Kumar, S., et al. "Effects of Serial Passage of Autographa Californiica Nuclear Polyhedrosis Virus in Cell Culture." *Virus Research,* 7 (1987), pp. 335-349.

777. See Note 774, p. 44.
778. Lederberg, J. *Science,* (October 20, 1967), p. 313.
779. See Note 774, p. 44.
780. Crow, T.J. "Is Schizophrenia an Infectious Disease?" *Lancet,* (1983), 1:8317, pp. 173-175.
781. Halonen, et al. "Antibody Levels to HSV-1, Measles, and Rubella Virus in Psychiatric Patients," *British Journal of Psychiatry,* 125 (1974), pp. 461-465.
782. Steinberg, D. et al, "Influenza Infection Causing Manic Psychosis," *British Journal of Psychiatry,* 120 (1972), pp. 531-535.
783. Morozov, P.V. ed., "Research on the Viral Hypothesis of Mental Disorders," *Advances in Biological Psychiatry,* Volume 12, (New York: S. Karger, 1983), pp. 52-75.
784. McGuire, R. "Brain Autoantibodies in 33% of Schizophrenics," *Medical Tribune,* (July 14, 1988), p. 6.
785. See Note 774, p. 44.
786. Leviton, R. "A Shot in the Dark," *Yoga Journal,* (May/June, 1992), pp. 112-114.
787. Bannister, R. *Brain's Clinical Neurology,* 5th Ed., (Oxford: University Press, 1978):409.
788. See Note 316, pp. xiii-xiv; Chapters 1-5.
789. See Note 316.
790. Ibid., p. 103.
791. Merritt, H.H. *Textbook of Neurology,* 6th Ed., (Philadelphia, PA:Lea and Febiger, 1979):104.
792. Neal, J.B. *Encephalitis: A Clinical Study,* (New York: Grune and Stratton, 1942), pp. 378-379.
793. See Note 791, pp. 102-103.
794. Ford, F.R. *Diseases of the Nervous System in Infancy, Childhood, and Adolescence,* (Springfield: C.C. Thomas, 1937), p. 349.
795. Lurie, et al. "Late Results Noted in Children Presenting Post-Encephalitic Behavior," *American Journal of Psychiatry,* 104, (1947), p. 178.
796. Baker, A.B. "The Central Nervous System in Infectious Diseases of Childhood,: *Postgraduate Medicine,* 5, (1949), p. 11.
797. Annell, A.L. "Pertussis in Infancy—A Cause of Behavioral Disorders in Children," *Acta Societatis Medicorum Upsaliensis,* XVIII, Supplement 1, (1953), pp. 17, 33.
798. See Notes 791 and 792.
799. See Note 316. pp. 120-121.
800. Kanner, L. "Autistic Disturbances of Affective Content," *The Nervous Child II,* (1942-1943), pp. 250.
801. American Psychiatric Association. *Diagnostic and Statistical Manual of Mental Disorders,* Third Edition, Revised, (Washington, DC, 1987), pp. 36-37.
802. Wakabayashi, S. "The Present Status of an Early Infantile Autism First Reported in Japan 30 Years Ago," *Nagoya Journal of Medical Science,* 1984; 46:35-39.
803. See Note 316, p. 50.
804. Ibid.
805. Kanner, L. "To What Extent is Early Infantile Autism Determined by Constitutional Inadequacies?" *Genetics and the Inheritance of Integrated Neurological and Psychiatric Patterns,* (Baltimore: Williams and Wilkins, 1954), p. 382.
806. Kanner, L., et al. "Early Infantile Autism: 1943-1955," *Psychiatric Research Reports,* 7 (1957): 62.
807. Kanner, L., "Early Infantile Autism," *Journal of Pediatrics,* 1944; 25:217.
808. Gillberg, C. and Schaumann, "Social Class and Infantile Autism," *Journal of Autism* 1982; 12(3), p. 223.
809. See Note 316, pp. 52-53.
810. "Autism: Present Challenges, Future Needs—Why the Increased Rates?" *Government Reform Committee Hearing,* Washington, DC. (April 6, 2000.) As cited in Chairman Dan Burton's opening statement.
811. Ibid. As cited in the testimony of Coleen Boyle, PhD.
812. See Note 810.
813. Wakefield, A.J., et al. "Ileal-lymphoid-nodular hyperplasia, non-specific colitis, and pervasive developmental disorder in children." *Lancet* 1998; 351:637-641.
814. Yazbak, F. E. "Autism: Is there a vaccine connection? Part I. Vaccination after delivery," 1999. www.garynull.com/documents/autism99b.htm "Part II. Vaccination around pregnancy," 1999. www.garynull.com/documents/autism99b2.htm "Part III. Vaccination around pregnancy, the sequel," 2000. www.garynull.com/documents/ autism99b3.htm
815. Yazbak, F. E., et al. "Adverse outcomes associated with postpartum rubella or MMR vaccine." *Medical Sentinel* 2001; 6(3):95-99,108.
816. Yazbak, F. E., et al. "Live virus vaccination near a pregnancy: flawed policies, tragic results." *Medical Hypotheses* (September 2002); 59(3):283-288.
817. Published by New Atlantean Press (Copyright © 2003; ISBN: 1-881217-32-9).
818. See Note 810.
819. Schilling, W. "VOSI research report RR8-V50.2." *Voices of Safety International (VOSI),* October 27, 2000. Research conclusions are based upon survey data analysis by Don Meserlian, VOSI chairman. www.voiceofsafety.com/t1-ph-v50-2-research-addendum.htm
820. See Note 262.
821. Ross, D.M., et al. *Hyperactivity: Research, Theory, and Action,* (New York: John Wiley, 1982).
822. Cowart, V.S. "Attention-Deficit Hyperactivity Disorder: Physicians Helping Parents Pay More Heed," *Journal of American Medical Association,* 259:18, (May 13, 1988), p. 2647.
823. Long, K. and Queen. "Detection and Treatment of Emotionally Disturbed Children in Public Schools: Problems and Theoretical Perspectives," *Journal of Clinical Psychology,* 40:1, (January 1984), p. 378.
824. See Note 822.

825. Healy, J.M. *Endangered Minds: Why Our Children Don't Think*, (New York: Simon & Schuster, Inc., 1990), pp. 13-15.
826. Ibid.
827. Ibid.
828. Ibid., pp. 17-18.
829. Ibid., pp. 27-35.
830. See Note 316, pp. 61-62.
831. Ibid., p. 112.
832. "Vaccine Fund Needs Booster Shot," *Common Cause Magazine*, (May/June, 1991), p. 10.
833. "Congress Votes Help to Youngster Hurt by Vaccine," *Tucson Citizen*, (May 9, 1990), p. 1-2A.
834. See Note 316, p. 113.
835. Ibid., p. 112.
836. "Vaccine-injured Girl Gets $2.4 Million," *Tampa Tribune*, (May 16, 1990), p. 1B.
837. See Note 316, pp. 179-181.
838. Bond, E.D. and Appel. *The Treatment of Behavior Disorders Following Encephalitis*, (New York: The Commonwealth Fund, 1931), p. 14-15.
839. Elliott, F.A. "Biological Roots of Violence," *Proceedings of the American Philosophical Society*, 127:2 (1983), pp. 84-93.
840. *The New York Times*, (December 5, 1987), p. B1.
841. Rimland, B. and Larson, "The Manpower Quality Decline: An Ecological Perspective," *Armed Forces and Society*, 8:1, (Fall 1981), p. 56.
842. See Note 316, pp. 186-187.
843. Lewis, D. ed., *Vulnerabilities to Delinquency*, (New York: SP Medical and Scientific Books, 1981), p. 28.
844. Hollander, H.E. and Turner. "Characteristics of Incarcerated Delinquents: Relationship Between Development Disorders, Environmental and Family Factors, and Patterns of Offense and Recidivism," *Journal of American Child Psychiatry*, 24:1, (1985), p. 225.
845. See Note 822.
846. Moyer, K.E. *The Psychobiology of Aggression*, (New York: Harper and Row, 1976), p. 36.
847. *Plan for a Nationwide Action on Epilepsy*, (Commission for the Control of Epilepsy, 1977), Volume 2, part 1, p. 822. (Unpublished material cited in Note 104, pp. 197-198.)
848. *The New York Times*, (September 17, 1985), p. C1+.
849. See Note 825, p. 140.
850. Lidsky, T.I., et al. "Are Movement Disorders the Most Serious Side Effects of Maintenance Therapy with Antipsychotic Drugs?" *Biological Psychiatry*, 16:12, (1981), pp. 1189-1194.
851. Cowart, V.S. "The Ritalin Controversy: What's Made This Drug's Opponents Hyperactive?" *Journal of the American Medical Association*, 259:17, (May 6, 1988), p. 2522.
852. Workman-Daniels, et al. "Childhood Problem Behavior and Neuropsychological Functioning in Persons at Risk for Alcoholism," *Journal of Studies on Alcoholism*, Volume 48:3, (1987), pp. 187-193.
853. Sarason, I.G., et al. *Abnormal Psychology*, Sixth Edition, (Englewood Cliffs, NJ: Prentice Hall, 1989), p. 433.
854. The National Childhood Vaccine Injury Act of 1986, Public Law 99-660, *The Compensation System and How it Works*. (National Vaccine Information Center, Vienna, VA., 1990), pp. 1-7.
855. See Note 319, pp. 7-10.
856. In a September 16, 1990 letter written by Barbara Loe Fisher, to Donald A. Henderson, chairman of the National Vaccine Advisory Committee, p. 3.
857. As reported in a National Vaccine Information Center press release. (Vienna, VA, January 27, 1999.)
858. Ibid.
859. *NVIC Mini News*. (Vienna, VA: National Vaccine Information Center, November 1990): 3.
860. *Vaccine Reaction Report*. (Vienna, VA: National Vaccine Information Center, November 25, 1991), pp. 23-24.
861. See Note 624, p. 34.
862. See Note 319, pp. 8-10.
863. Barkin and Pichichero. "Diphtheria-pertussis-tetanus vaccine: Reactogenicity of commercial products," *Pediatrics*, 63:2, (February 2, 1979), pp. 256-260.
864. See Note 314, pp. 55-56.
865. See Note 765, p. 19.
866. Institute of Medicine. *Vaccine Safety Committee Proceedings* (National Academy of Sciences: Washington, DC, May 11, 1992), pp. 93-105.
867. *NVIC Mini News*. (Vienna, VA: National Vaccine Information Center, March 1991): 1.
868. In a February 25, 1991 letter written by Jeffrey H. Schwartz of NVIC, to Walter A. Orenstein, M.D., director of the Division of Immunization, CDC, with accompanying *Comments on Proposed Vaccine Information Materials*. In a March 13, 1991 letter to Dr. Claire Broome of the CDC, with accompanying appendices.
869. See Note 856, p. 1.
870. Ibid., p. 2.
871. In a May 8, 1991 letter written by Jeffrey H. Schwartz of NVIC, to Louis M. Sullivan, secretary of the Department of Health and Human Services. In a May 9, 1991 press release issued by NVIC.
872. "Conflicts of Interest and Vaccine Development: Preserving the Integrity of the Process." *Government Reform Committee Hearing*, Washington, DC. (June 15, 2000.) As cited in Chairman Dan Burton's opening statement.
873. Ibid.
874. Ibid.

875. CDC. "Withdrawal of rotavirus vaccine recommendation." *MMWR Weekly* (November 5, 1999); 48(43):1007.

876. Congressional Press Release. "Burton critical of vaccine approval process: staff report details FDA and CDC conflicts in approval of controversial rotavirus vaccine." *Committee on Government Reform* (August 23, 2000).

877. Mitchell, S. "Congressional report slams FDA, CDC policies on disclosing financial conflicts." *Reuters Medical News* (August 24, 2000).

878. Ibid.

879. Ibid.

880. See Note 39.

881. "Why am I so sick?" *20-20 Newscast*, (January 26, 1990).

882. "Concerned parents unfairly shut out of congressional hearings on vaccines," *Dayton Daily News* (May 28, 1993), p. 15A.

883. See Note 866, pp. 40-41.

884. Kessler, D.A. "Introducing MEDWatch: A New Approach to Reporting Medication and Device Adverse Effects and Product Problems," *Journal of American Medical Association* (June 2, 1993), p. 2765.

885. National Vaccine Injury Compensation Program. "Monthly statistics report." (Awards paid through November 10, 1999.)

886. See Note 854.

887. Hilts, P.J. "U.S. vaccine plan uses welfare offices." *New York Times* (March 17, 1991), p. 26.

888. Dixon, J. "$25 in Welfare Rides on Children's Shots," *Los Angeles Times* (June 27, 1993).

889. As communicated to the author during several telephone conversations.

890. See Note 765, pp. 131-146.

891. Goodwin, Jan. "Murder or vaccine?" *Redbook* (September 2000), p. 159.

892. Hickman, Maureen. "Shaken baby syndrome or adverse vaccine reaction?" *Nexus New Times* (November-December, 2000), pp. 33+.

893. Scheibner, Viera. "Shaken baby syndrome—the vaccination link." *Nexus* (August-September, 1998), pp. 35+.

894. *Vaccine Reaction Report,* (Vienna, VA: National Vaccine Information Center, November 25, 1991), pp. 23-24.

895. Airola, Paavo. "Immunization: A New Look," *Everywoman's Book,* (Phoenix, AZ: Health Plus, 1979), pp. 271-285.

896. See Note 23, p. 142.

897. McBean, Eleanor Ph.D., *Vaccinations Do Not Protect,* (Manachaca, TX: Health Excellence Systems, 1991), pp. 13-14.

898. Hume, E. Douglas. *Bechamp or Pasteur,* (Mokelumne Hill, CA: Health Research, 1989). Abridged reprint by Health Research.

899. Sheehan, Michael. "Was Pasteur Wrong?" *Natural Health* (Jan/Feb 1992), pp. 41-44.

900. Ibid.

901. See Note 898.

902. Savage, Patricia. "A Mother's Research on Immunizations," *Mothering* (Fall 1979), p. 79.

903. See Note 895, pp. 285-287.

904. See Note 765, pp. 195-197: Appendix A—Keys to a Healthy Immune System, A Holistic Approach.

905. See Note 23, p. 9.

906. See Note 143, p. 31.

907. Weiss, R. "Breastmilk may stimulate immunity," *Science News* (March 26, 1988), p. 196.

908. Grossman, Lindsey. "Breastfeeding healthier babies," *USA Today* (August 1988), p. 4.

909. Cunningham, Allan. "Breastfeeding and health," *The Compleat Mother* (Summer 1987), p. 36.

910. See Note 334.

911. Manahan, William. *Eat For Health* (Tiburon, CA: H.J. Kramer, Inc., 1988), pp. 60-76.

912. See Note 186, pp. 54-55.

913. Ibid., pp. 163-165.

914. "Is a 'Gimmick' the Answer?" *AMA News* (Feb. 1, 1985), pp. 1+.

915. "Stars Say 'Get Your Shots!'" *Weekly Reader* (Feb. 21, 1992), p. 1.

916. Moskowitz, Richard. "Vaccination: A Sacrament of Modern Medicine." Presented in a speech at the Annual Conference of the Society of Homeopaths, (Manchester, England, September 1991).

Index

Purchasing Information

Additional copies of **Vaccines: Are They *Really* Safe and Effective?** (ISBN: 1-881217-30-2) may be purchased directly from *New Atlantean Press*. Call 505-983-1856. Or send $12.95 (in U.S. funds), plus $3.50 shipping, to:

New Atlantean Press
PO Box 9638
Santa Fe, NM 87504
505-983-1856 (Telephone & Fax)
Email: global@thinktwice.com

This book is also available at many fine bookstores and health stores. Be sure to inform the sales clerk that you want the *revised* edition: 1-881217-30-2.

Bookstores and Retail Buyers: Order from Baker & Taylor, Ingram, Midpoint, New Leaf, Nutri-Books, or from New Atlantean Press. Libraries may order this book from Quality Books, Unique Books, or from your favorite library wholesaler.

Chiropractors, Homeopaths, Midwives, Naturopaths, Pediatricians, Vaccine Organizations, and other Non-Storefront Buyers: Take a 40% discount with the purchase of 5 or more copies (multiply the total cost of purchases x .60). Please add 7% ($3.50 minimum) for shipping.

Shipping: Please add 7% ($3.50 minimum) for shipping. Allow one to three weeks for your order to arrive, or include $3.00 extra for priority air mail shipping. **Foreign orders** must include 20% ($5.50 minimum) for shipping. Air mail is available. Please email us for rates: global@thinktwice.com Checks must be drawn on a U.S. bank, or send a Postal Money Order in U.S. funds. **Sales Tax:** Please add 6% for books shipped to New Mexico addresses.

Vaccine Laws: A copy of the vaccine laws of YOUR state are now available. Don't allow yourself to be intimidated by overzealous authorities. Arm yourself with the exact laws of your state. Code VSL: $4 (specify state).

Sample Exemption Letter: Do you wish to exempt your child from vaccines? You must create an exemption letter that conforms to state law. This 2-page kit includes a sample exemption letter and recommendations. Code SAU: $4.

FREE CATALOG: *New Atlantean Press* offers the world's largest selection of uncensored vaccine information, including up-to-date vaccine laws, vaccine books, and other hard-to-find vaccine resources. We also offer numerous books on cutting-edge alternative health solutions, natural immunity, progressive parenting, holistic childcare, AIDS, cancer, and more. Send for a free catalog: *New Atlantean Press*, PO Box 9638, Santa Fe, NM 87504. Or visit the:

Thinktwice Global Vaccine Institute
www.thinktwice.com

Neil Z. Miller is a medical research journalist and natural health advocate. He is the author of numerous articles and books on vaccines, and is the director of the *Thinktwice Global Vaccine Institute*. He has a degree in psychology (with an emphasis on statistical analysis) and is a member of Mensa. He lives in Northern New Mexico with his family.

What others are saying about this book:

"Neil Miller is making a transformative contribution to the world with this book on vaccines—a mindful, liberating work to be a classic in the holistic health literature. Hygieia's highest recommendation to everyone who loves children and the future of our planet."—Jeannine Parvati Baker, Director, Hygieia College, Midwife, Childbirth Educator, and author of *Hygieia Herbal, Conscious Conception,* and *Prenatal Yoga*

"Mr. Miller points out the dangers of the 'mandatory' vaccines and of several others. His descriptions of each illness and delineation of the controversy are noteworthy."—American Library Association Booklist

"Compelling evidence! This book deeply affected me. I strongly recommend it to all concerned parents."—Rayna Siegler-Dineen, MA, Early Childhood Educator

"This book on vaccines should be read by every parent and every health professional. I only wish it had been available when my wife and I had to make the difficult decision of whether or not to vaccinate our daughter."—Marvin Surkin, PhD, Natural Health Practitioner

"I have read your book on vaccines and was deeply moved and extremely appreciative."—Christine Ostic, Concerned Parent

"The book was a 'Mind Blower.' Thank you."—Jean Stewart, New Mom

"Your book is excellent—I'm spreading the word!"—Cynthia Goldenberg, Concerned Mother, whose once healthy son is now autistic as a result of the MMR vaccine

"There is a growing controversy on this subject and Mr. Miller needs to be heard."—George R. Schwartz, MD, Physician, Toxicologist, and Senior Editor of *Principles and Practice of Emergency Medicine*

"Congratulations! Finally there is something to give patients when they inquire about this overwhelming conundrum. I've already told many people about this important contribution."—Janet Zand, ND, Doctor of Naturopathy, Oriental Medicine, and Certified Acupuncturist

"This book is a must for all who have, or are contemplating having, children."—NAPRA Trade Journal

"A growing number of people are refusing to have their children immunized. Mr. Miller believes this issue is about to explode."—The Boston Herald

"There are grounds for questioning both the safety and efficacy of current childhood vaccination programs. These reasons are reviewed with clarity and thoroughness in the main body of this book."—Harold E. Buttram, MD

*This book is dedicated
to parents and children
everywhere.*